Treatment of Lower Urinary Tract Symptoms and Benign Prostatic Hyperplasia

Editors

KEVIN T. MCVARY
CHARLES WELLIVER

UROLOGIC CLINICS OF NORTH AMERICA

www.urologic.theclinics.com

Consulting Editor
SAMIR S. TANEJA

August 2016 • Volume 43 • Number 3

ELSEVIER

1600 John F. Kennedy Boulevard • Suite 1800 • Philadelphia, Pennsylvania, 19103-2899

http://www.theclinics.com

UROLOGIC CLINICS OF NORTH AMERICA Volume 43, Number 3
August 2016 ISSN 0094-0143, ISBN-13: 978-0-323-45993-8

Editor: Kerry Holland
Developmental Editor: Alison Swety

Urologic Clinics of North America (ISSN 0094-0143) is published quarterly by Elsevier Inc., 360 Park Avenue South, New York, NY 10010-1710. Months of issue are February, May, August, and November. Business and Editorial Offices: 1600 John F. Kennedy Blvd., Suite 1800, Philadelphia, PA 19103-2899. Periodicals postage paid at New York, NY and additional mailing offices. Subscription prices are $360.00 per year (US individuals), $660.00 per year (US institutions), $415.00 per year (Canadian individuals), $825.00 per year (Canadian institutions), $515.00 per year (foreign individuals), and $825.00 per year (foreign institutions). Foreign air speed delivery is included in all *Clinics* subscription prices. All prices are subject to change without notice. **POSTMASTER:** Send address changes to *Urologic Clinics of North America*, Elsevier Health Sciences Division, Subscription Customer Service, 3251 Riverport Lane, Maryland Heights, MO 63043. **Customer Service: 1-800-654-2452 (US). From outside the United States, call 1-314-447-8871. Fax: 1-314-447-8029. E-mail: JournalsCustomerServiceusa@elsevier.com (for print support)** and **JournalsOnlineSupport-usa@elsevier.com (for online support)**.

Reprints. For copies of 100 or more, of articles in this publication, please contact the Commercial Reprints Department, Elsevier Inc., 360 Park Avenue South, New York, New York 10010-1710. Tel.: 212-633-3874; Fax: 212-633-3820; E-mail: reprints@elsevier.com.

Urologic Clinics of North America is covered in MEDLINE/PubMed (*Index Medicus*), *Excerpta Medica, Current Contents/Clinical Medicine, Science Citation Index,* and *ISI/BIOMED.*

PROGRAM OBJECTIVE

The goal of *Urologic Clinics of North America* is to keep practicing urologists and urology residents up to date with current clinical practice in urology by providing timely articles reviewing the state of the art in patient care.

TARGET AUDIENCE

Practicing urologists, urology residents and other health care professionals practicing in the discipline of urology.

LEARNING OBJECTIVES

Upon completion of this activity, participants will be able to:
1. Review the diagnostic workup for and treatments for lower urinary tract symptoms.
2. Discuss the use of pharmaceuticals in the medical management of lower urinary tract symptoms and benign prostatic hyperplasia.
3. Recognize potential side effects of medical and surgical treatments for benign prostatic hyperplasia.

ACCREDITATION

The Elsevier Office of Continuing Medical Education (EOCME) is accredited by the Accreditation Council for Continuing Medical Education (ACCME) to provide continuing medical education for physicians.

The EOCME designates this enduring material for a maximum of 15 *AMA PRA Category 1 Credit*(s)™. Physicians should claim only the credit commensurate with the extent of their participation in the activity.

All other health care professionals requesting continuing education credit for this enduring material will be issued a certificate of participation.

DISCLOSURE OF CONFLICTS OF INTEREST

The EOCME assesses conflict of interest with its instructors, faculty, planners, and other individuals who are in a position to control the content of CME activities. All relevant conflicts of interest that are identified are thoroughly vetted by EOCME for fair balance, scientific objectivity, and patient care recommendations. EOCME is committed to providing its learners with CME activities that promote improvements or quality in healthcare and not a specific proprietary business or a commercial interest.

The planning committee, staff, authors and editors listed below have identified no financial relationships or relationships to products or devices they or their spouse/life partner have with commercial interest related to the content of this CME activity:

LaTayia Aaron, BS; Reem Aldamanhori, MD, MBBS, SB-Urol; Christopher R. Chapple, BSc, MD, FRCS (Urol), FEBU; Kenneth Jackson DeLay, MD; Kathryn Brigham Egan, PhD, MPH; Ahmed Essa, MD; Anjali Fortna; Omar E. Franco, MD, PhD; Claudius Füllhase, MD, PhD; Simon W. Hayward, PhD; Sarah L. Hecht, MD; Jason C. Hedges, MD, PhD; Marc Holden, MD; Kerry Holland; Indu Kumari; Herbert Lepor, MD; Nadir I. Osman, MBChB (Hons), PhD, MRCS; J. Kellogg Parsons, MD, MHS; Marc P. Schneider, MD; Megan Suermann; Dominique Thomas, BS.

The planning committee, staff, authors and editors listed below have identified financial relationships or relationships to products or devices they or their spouse/life partner have with commercial interest related to the content of this CME activity:

Bilal Chughtai, MD is a consultant/advisor for Boston Scientific Corporation.
Jean-Nicolas Cornu, MD, PhD, FEBU is a consultant/advisor for Bouchora Recordati; Astellas Pharma US; Allergan; and Boston Scientific Corporation.
Steven Kaplan, MD is a consultant/advisor for, with research support from, Astellas Pharma US.
Tobias S. Kohler, MD is a consultant/advisor for Coloplast Corp; Boston Scientific Corporation; Abbvie Inc.; and Lipocine Inc., and has research support from Coloplast Corp; Boston Scientific Corporation; and AbbVie Inc.
Altaf Mangera, MBChB, MD, FRCS (Urol) is on the speakers' bureau for Astellas Pharma US.
Kevin T. McVary, MD, FACS is a consultant/advisor for Eli Lilly and Company, and has research support from The National Institute of Diabetes and Digestive and Kidney Diseases; Astellas Pharma US; Boston Scientific Corporation; and Sophiris Bio, Corp.
Claus G. Roehrborn, MD is a consultant/advisor for, with research support from, NeoTract, Inc.
Samir S. Taneja, MD is a consultant/advisor for Bayer HealthCare Pharmaceuticals; Eigen Pharma LLC, GTx, Inc.; Health-Tronics, Inc.; and Hitachi, Ltd.
Charles Welliver, MD is a consultant/advisor for Coloplast Corp, with research support from Capital Region Medical Research Foundation, and receives royalties/patents from Oakstone and BMJ Publishing Group Limited.

UNAPPROVED/OFF-LABEL USE DISCLOSURE

The EOCME requires CME faculty to disclose to the participants:
1. When products or procedures being discussed are off-label, unlabelled, experimental, and/or investigational (not US Food and Drug Administration [FDA] approved); and

2. Any limitations on the information presented, such as data that are preliminary or that represent ongoing research, interim analyses, and/or unsupported opinions. Faculty may discuss information about pharmaceutical agents that is outside of FDA-approved labelling. This information is intended solely for CME and is not intended to promote off-label use of these medications. If you have any questions, contact the medical affairs department of the manufacturer for the most recent prescribing information.

TO ENROLL
To enroll in the *Urologic Clinics of North America* Continuing Medical Education program, call customer service at 1-800-654-2452 or sign up online at http://www.theclinics.com/home/cme. The CME program is available to subscribers for an additional annual fee of USD $270.

METHOD OF PARTICIPATION
In order to claim credit, participants must complete the following:
1. Complete enrolment as indicated above.
2. Read the activity.
3. Complete the CME Test and Evaluation. Participants must achieve a score of 70% on the test. All CME Tests and Evaluations must be completed online.

CME INQUIRIES/SPECIAL NEEDS
For all CME inquiries or special needs, please contact elsevierCME@elsevier.com.

Contributors

CONSULTING EDITOR

SAMIR S. TANEJA, MD
The James M. Neissa and Janet Riha Neissa
Professor of Urologic Oncology; Professor of
Urology and Radiology; Director, Division of
Urologic Oncology; Co-Director, Department
of Urology, Smilow Comprehensive Prostate
Cancer Center, NYU Langone Medical Center,
New York, New York

EDITORS

KEVIN T. McVARY, MD, FACS
Professor and Chair, Division of Urology,
Southern Illinois University School of Medicine,
Springfield, Illinois

CHARLES WELLIVER, MD
Assistant Professor, Division of Urology,
Albany Medical College; Staff Physician,
Albany Stratton Veterans Affairs Medical
Center; Urological Institute of Northeastern
New York, Albany, New York

AUTHORS

LATAYIA AARON, BS
Graduate Student, Department of
Biochemistry and Cancer Biology, Meharry
Medical College, Nashville, Tennessee;
Department of Surgery, NorthShore University
HealthSystem Research Institute, Evanston,
Illinois

REEM ALDAMANHORI, MD, MBBS, SB-Urol
Assistant Professor, University of Dammam,
Khobar, Kingdom of Saudi Arabia; Urology
Registrar, Royal Hallamshire Hospital,
Sheffield, United Kingdom

**CHRISTOPHER R. CHAPPLE, BSc, MD,
FRCS (Urol), FEBU**
Professor, Department of Urology, Royal
Hallamshire Hospital, Sheffield, United
Kingdom

BILAL CHUGHTAI, MD
Assistant Professor of Urology, Department
of Urology, Weill Cornell Medicine-New York,
Presbyterian Hospital, New York,
New York

JEAN-NICOLAS CORNU, MD, PhD, FEBU
Department of Urology, Rouen University
Hospital, University of Rouen, Rouen,
France

KENNETH JACKSON DELAY, MD
Department of Urology, Tulane University
Health Sciences Center, New Orleans,
Louisiana

KATHRYN BRIGHAM EGAN, PhD, MPH
Yale University, New Haven, Connecticut;
New England Research Institutes Inc.,
Watertown, Massachusetts

AHMED ESSA, MD
University of Al - Iraqi School of Medicine;
Department of Urology, Al-Numan Teaching
Hospital, Baghdad, Iraq

OMAR E. FRANCO, MD, PhD
Research Scientist II, Department of Surgery,
NorthShore University HealthSystem Research
Institute, Evanston, Illinois

CLAUDIUS FÜLLHASE, MD, PhD
Department of Urology, University of Rostock, Rostock, Germany

SIMON W. HAYWARD, PhD
Adjunct Professor, Department of Biochemistry and Cancer Biology, Meharry Medical College, Nashville, Tennessee; Jean Ruggles Romoser Chair of Cancer Research and Director of Cancer Biology, Department of Surgery, NorthShore University HealthSystem Research Institute, Evanston, Illinois

SARAH L. HECHT, MD
Urology Resident, Urology, Oregon Health and Science University, Portland, Oregon

JASON C. HEDGES, MD, PhD
Assistant Professor, Urology, Oregon Health and Science University, Portland, Oregon

MARC HOLDEN, MD
Moores Cancer Center, University of California at San Diego, San Diego, California

STEVEN KAPLAN, MD
Department of Urology, Mount Sinai Hospital, New York, New York

TOBIAS S. KOHLER, MD
Division of Urology, Southern Illinois University School of Medicine, Springfield, Illinois

HERBERT LEPOR, MD
Urologist in Chief, NYU Langone Medical Center, Professor and Martin Spatz Chair of Urology, NYU School of Medicine, New York, New York

ALTAF MANGERA, MBChB, MD, FRCS (Urol)
Urology Resident, Department of Urology, Royal Hallamshire Hospital, Sheffield, United Kingdom

KEVIN T. McVARY, MD, FACS
Professor and Chair, Division of Urology, Southern Illinois University School of Medicine, Springfield, Illinois

NADIR I. OSMAN, MBChB (Hons), PhD, MRCS
Urology Resident, Department of Urology, Royal Hallamshire Hospital, Sheffield, United Kingdom

J. KELLOGG PARSONS, MD, MHS
Associate Professor of Surgery, Moores Cancer Center, University of California at San Diego, San Diego, California

CLAUS G. ROEHRBORN, MD
Professor and Chairman, Department of Urology, UT Southwestern Medical Center, Dallas, Texas

MARC P. SCHNEIDER, MD
Department of Health Science and Technology, Swiss Federal Institute of Technology Zurich, Brain Research Institute, University of Zurich, Zurich, Switzerland

DOMINIQUE THOMAS, BS
Department of Urology, Weill Cornell Medicine-New York, Presbyterian Hospital, New York, New York

CHARLES WELLIVER, MD
Assistant Professor, Division of Urology, Albany Medical College; Staff Physician, Albany Stratton Veterans Affairs Medical Center; Urological Institute of Northeastern New York, Albany, New York

Contents

Prostate development follows a common pattern between species and depends on the actions of androgens to induce and support ductal branching morphogenesis of buds emerging from the urogenital sinus. The human prostate has a compact zonal anatomy immediately surrounding the urethra and below the urinary bladder. Rodents have a lobular prostate with lobes radiating away from the urethra. The human prostate is the site of benign hyperplasia, prostate cancer, and prostatitis. The rodent prostate has little naturally occurring disease. Rodents can be used to model aspects of human benign hyperplasia, but care should be taken in data interpretation and extrapolation to the human condition.

This article assesses the reported prevalence and incidence rates for benign prostatic hyperplasia and lower urinary tract symptoms (BPH/LUTS) by age, symptom severity, and race/ethnicity. BPH/LUTS prevalence and incidence rates increase with age and vary by symptom severity. The BPH/LUTS relationship is complex due to several factors. This contributes to the range of reported estimates and difficulties in drawing epidemiologic comparisons. Cultural, psychosocial, economic, and/or disease awareness and diagnosis factors may influence medical care access, symptom reporting, and help-seeking behaviors among men with BPH/LUTS. However, these factors and their epidemiologic association with BPH/LUTS have not been thoroughly investigated.

The goal of work-up of lower urinary tract symptoms is to establish the severity and cause of lower urinary tract symptoms and to predict with certainty which patients will respond to which treatments. Clinical guidelines exist to guide urologists in decision-making. All patients need a medical history with a validated symptom score, a physical examination, and a urinalysis. Prostate-specific antigen, postvoid urine residual, and peak urine flow rate provide additional information at little cost. For more invasive testing high-level data are lacking and guidelines defer to the urologist. Even the most extensive work-up is imperfect, and thus the attempt to balance costs with benefits of invasive testing.

Treatments for lower urinary tract symptoms due to benign prostatic hyperplasia can be evaluated by multiple metrics. A balance within the confines of patient expectations is key to determining the ideal treatment. A troubling adverse event for some patients is sexual dysfunction. Because the cohort of men who seek treatment of sexual dysfunction and lower urinary tract symptoms is essentially identical, these disease processes frequently overlap. This article considers potential pathophysiologic causes of dysfunction with treatment and attempts to critically review the available data to assess the true incidence of sexual adverse events with treatment.

Despite a lack of evidence, there have been stated concerns that testosterone replacement therapy (TRT) can pose a risk to men suffering with lower urinary tract symptoms (LUTS)/benign prostatic hyperplasia (BPH). TRT may improve components of the metabolic syndrome, which is associated with worsening LUTS. Furthermore, the evidence suggests that TRT may decrease prostatic inflammation, which is also associated with worsening LUTS. The data on the relationship between TRT and LUTS have never shown worsening of LUTS, often show no change in LUTS, and occasionally show improvement.

UROLOGIC CLINICS OF NORTH AMERICA

THE CLINICS ARE AVAILABLE ONLINE!
Access your subscription at:
www.theclinics.com

UROLOGIC CLINICS OF NORTH AMERICA

FORTHCOMING ISSUES

November 2016
Penile, Urethral, and Scrotal Cancer
Philippe E. Spiess, Editor

February 2017
Male Urethral Reconstruction and the Management of Urethral Stricture Disease
Lee C. Zhao, Editor

May 2017
Small Renal Mass
Alexander Kutikov and Marc Smaldone, Editors

RECENT ISSUES

May 2016
Hypogonadism
Joseph P. Alukal, Editor

February 2016
Biomarkers in Urologic Cancer
Kevin R. Loughlin, Editor

November 2015
Contemporary Antibiotic Management for Urologic Procedures and Infections
Sarah C. Flury and Anthony J. Schaeffer, Editors

Foreword
Treatment of Lower Urinary Tract Symptoms and Benign Prostatic Hyperplasia

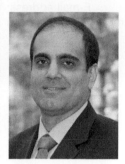

Samir S. Taneja, MD
Consulting Editor

Since the initiation of Urology as a surgical specialty, the surgical management of benign prostatic hyperplasia (BPH) has been a mainstay of practice. As an inevitable process of aging, the severity of lower urinary tract symptoms associated with aging varies greatly, perhaps owing to a more complex physiology than just mechanical obstruction due to a big gland. The historical evolution of technologies related to the surgical treatment of BPH is fascinating and is perhaps one of the greatest testimonials for the obsession of urologists with devices and mechanical tools. From the days of open simple perineal prostatectomies, to the current state-of-the-art laser techniques, the impact of such surgical techniques on our patient's quality of life remains immense.

A number of factors have influenced the utilization of surgery in the management of BPH over the past many years. As a medical student, I watched my residents perform score after score of transurethral resections as part of their training. By the time I was a resident in the early 1990s, the use of transurethral resection was on the decline, in part due to the rapid uptick of radical prostatectomy in the prostate-specific antigen screening era, and, in part, due to the development of medical therapies by pioneers

like my eventual Chair and mentor, Herb Lepor. In the present day, the management of BPH is completely changed as compared with the days of my training. Pharmacologic management is evolved to include specific targeted agents related to both the nature of prostate obstruction and the degree of associated bladder dysfunction. Surgical management has survived despite the pharmacologic advances, largely because of the desire of patients to have definitive resolution and the inevitable progression of the disease, despite drug therapy. Current surgical therapy has far less morbidity than the techniques of previous generations, but has become more complex given the multitude of potential technologies that can be employed, the necessary skill associated with each technique, and the more rigorous measures of success or failure.

In this issue of *Urologic Clinics*, we review the current state-of-the-art in managing lower urinary tract symptoms associated with BPH. Our guest editors, Drs Kevin T. McVary and Charles Welliver, have picked the most contemporary topics for the reader's consideration and review. It is my sense that the management of BPH is largely driven by operator experience, preference, and access to individual

Urol Clin N Am 43 (2016) xiii–xiv
http://dx.doi.org/10.1016/j.ucl.2016.06.002
0094-0143/16/$ – see front matter © 2016 Published by Elsevier Inc.

urologic.theclinics.com

technologies. It is my hope that issues such as this one will help our readers to develop a more evidence-based algorithm for both surgery and medical therapy in the management of their patients, thereby improving outcomes across the board. I am deeply indebted to Drs McVary and Welliver, and to the individual authors of each outstanding article, for their hard work and dedication in the preparation of this issue of *Urologic Clinics*.

Samir S. Taneja, MD
Division of Urologic Oncology
Smilow Comprehensive Prostate Cancer Center
Department of Urology
NYU Langone Medical Center
150 East 32nd Street, Suite 200
New York, NY 10016, USA

E-mail address:
samir.taneja@nyumc.org

Preface

CrossMark

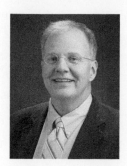
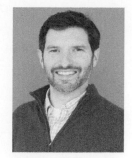

Kevin T. McVary, MD, FACS   Charles Welliver, MD

Editors

If there is any disease or surgical procedure that epitomizes urology to the public, then it is certainly the surgical treatment of benign prostatic disease. How many of us became "ureteral buds" upon entering our first operating room and witnessing the controlled chaos of wet floors, streams of blood on surgical gowns, and bombastic voices that (hopefully) culminated in a catheter-free and grateful older gentleman?

That very real vision was benign prostatic hyperplasia (BPH) treatment not so long ago. Our field and the options for our patients have expanded greatly in the past 20 years, in part to the efforts of many of the authors found in this series. Our patients can be managed medically, minimally invasively, and more traditionally with approaches tailored to their own phenotypes—a movement toward personalized medicine. Novel diagnostic tools, new treatments and methods for treatment delivery, modern surgical techniques, and a better understanding of the psychological and biological forces that drive lower urinary tract symptoms (LUTS) are bound to improve outcomes for our patients.

All of medicine is under pressure from outside forces. The treatment of LUTS/BPH is particularly under such intense scrutiny because medical treatments are common and costly, while the surgeries are numerous and potentially duplicative. These negative influences on this field are offset by the profound good our efforts obtain. Ask yourself as a surgeon, is there any more grateful patient than a previously catheter-dependent or home-bound man who gets effective treatment and now rejoins the world feeling significantly better? A numbers-needed-to-treat analysis of

N = 1! These appreciative patients, the increasing diverse choices for medications, the rapidly evolving technology, and the means to measure our impact on patients makes the field of LUTS/BPH boundlessly rewarding.

The contributors of the articles herein are not only recognized international leaders in the treatment of LUTS/BPH but also dedicated global instructors that put forth dedicated efforts to make this issue a reality. We are indebted to their support and efforts. We also express our appreciation to Dr Samir S. Taneja for supporting this endeavor and to Kerry Holland, Remy Van Wyk, Alison Swety, and Susan Showalter at Elsevier for their guidance throughout the process. Our hope is that the readers find this to be an engaging and informative issue.

In closing, we would like to thank our mentors, families, and patients. We could not be the physicians and people that we are without the impact all of these people have had on us.

Kevin T. McVary, MD, FACS
Southern Illinois University
School of Medicine
301 North 8th Street
Springfield, IL 62702, USA

Charles Welliver, MD
Albany Medical College
23 Hackett Boulevard
Albany, NY 12208, USA

E-mail addresses:
kmcvary@siumed.edu (K.T. McVary)
cwelliver@communitycare.com (C. Welliver)

Urol Clin N Am 43 (2016) xv
http://dx.doi.org/10.1016/j.ucl.2016.06.001
0094-0143/16/$ – see front matter © 2016 Published by Elsevier Inc.

Review of Prostate Anatomy and Embryology and the Etiology of Benign Prostatic Hyperplasia

LaTayia Aaron, BS[a,b], Omar E. Franco, MD, PhD[b],
Simon W. Hayward, PhD[a,b],*

KEYWORDS

- Prostate embryology • Prostate anatomy • BPH • LUTS

KEY POINTS

- Development of the prostate in humans and laboratory animals follows similar principles but the details vary.
- The anatomy of the human prostate is significantly different from that seen in laboratory animals.
- The disease profile of the human and rodent prostate is very different.
- Animal models describe certain aspects of human BPH but not the whole disease profile.
- Care should be taken in extrapolating observations made in rodents and applying them to humans.

INTRODUCTION

The human prostate is a walnut-sized organ at the base of the urinary bladder. It is the seat of three major causes of morbidity: (1) benign prostatic hyperplasia (BPH), (2) prostate cancer, and (3) prostatitis. As such it commands more attention than might be expected from an organ of this size. Anatomic illustrations of the prostate have been published dating at least as far back as the mid-sixteenth century when Andreas Vesalius, in 1543, published his observations of the male accessory glands.[1] The links between testicular and prostatic function have also been known for hundreds of years. John Hunter, writing in 1786 in "Observations on the glands situated between the rectum and the bladder, called vesiculae

seminales" said "the prostate and Cowper's glands and those of the urethra which in the perfect male are soft and bulky with a secretion salty to the taste, in the castrated animal are small, flabby, tough and ligermentous and have little secretion."[2]

The adult prostate is a compound tubular-alveolar gland found in most mammals.[3] The gross structure differs considerably between species. Much of the descriptive work on the development of the prostate from its origins in the hindgut to descriptions of the adult organ was performed by anatomists and pathologists working in the early to mid-twentieth century. Subsequent work has outlined the molecular basis for these descriptions. Interest in prostate biology is centered around the human organ and that of the species, notably rats

Disclosure Statement: The authors have nothing to disclose.
This work was supported in part by National Institutes of Health grants 1R01 DK103483 and 2 R25 GM059994-13.
[a] Department of Biochemistry and Cancer Biology, Meharry Medical College, 1005 DR DB Todd JR Blvd, Nashville, TN 37208, USA; [b] Department of Surgery, NorthShore University HealthSystem Research Institute, 1001 University Place, Evanston, IL 60201, USA
* Corresponding author. Cancer Biology, NorthShore University HealthSystem Research Institute, 1001 University Place, Evanston, IL 60201.
E-mail address: shayward@northshore.org

urologic.theclinics.com

and mice, used to model human diseases. A clear understanding of the differences in the structure of human and rodent prostates is important in assessing the results of animal studies.

HUMAN AND RODENT PROSTATE EMBRYOLOGY AND POSTNATAL DEVELOPMENT

The early mammalian embryo has the potential to develop toward a male or female phenotype. In genetically normal individuals this course is determined at conception and is reflected at the embryonic stage by the interactions of four critical units: (1) the wolffian duct, (2) the müllerian duct, (3) the urogenital sinus (UGS), and (4) the fetal gonad.

In humans the wolffian ducts start to develop approximately 25 to 30 days after conception in 2- to 3-mm-long embryos. These ducts initially act as excretory canals for the mesonephros, which performs the renal function in the early embryo. The ducts do not become incorporated into the genital system until the excretory function has been taken over by the definitive kidney. The ureters are a diverticulm of the wolffian duct, which becomes separated from the genital tract structures during development and which is the only part of the wolffian duct–derived structures that is preserved in the adult female. In such species as birds and reptiles, where the mesonephros has a prolonged excretory function, the wolffian ducts are preserved in an ambisexual state, in some cases until birth. In the human, by the time the embryo has reached 4 to 5 mm the ducts have elongated and lumenized to link the hindgut (which caudally becomes the cloaca) with the mesonephros and gonad.

The müllerian ducts develop later than the wolffian ducts, at about 6 weeks of gestation. A cleft lined with epithelial cells is formed between the gonadal and mesonephric parts of the urogenital ridge. This closes to form a tube that then extends through the surrounding mesenchyme parallel to the wolffian ducts. By the eighth week of gestation the müllerian ducts, which by this time are between the wolffian ducts, reach (but do not break into) the UGS forming the müllerian tubercule.

The UGS is produced in the 7- to 9-mm embryo by the formation of the urorectal septum, which divides the cloaca into the rectum and the UGS. The upper part of the UGS forms the urethra, whereas the part below the müllerian tubercule forms part of the vagina in the female and the penile urethra in the male.

The process of male sexual differentiation is determined under the influence of androgens produced by the fetal testis. In the absence of either these hormones or appropriate receptors, because of either an absent testis, lack of testicular function, or a mutation in the androgen receptor gene, the fetus develops a female phenotype. In the male, sexual differentiation is an asymmetric process consisting of the regression of the müllerian duct system, under the influence of Anti-Müllerian hormone expressed in the testicular Sertoli cells and stabilization, by androgens, of the wolffian ducts.

The second part of male sexual differentiation occurs under the influence of testosterone produced by the Leydig cells of the fetal testis. This involves changes in the tubules connecting the testis with the mesonephros to form the vasa efferentia, the formation of the convoluted epididymal duct and the vas deferens. The androgenic stimulus also acts to masculinize the UGS and the external genitalia. This process involves the formation of the prostate and the prostatic utricle, the closure of the labial-scrotal lobes, and the formation of the penis.

The rudimentary prostate starts to appear in 50-mm human embryos as epithelial buds growing laterally from the walls of the UGS at the site of the müllerian tubercle. Under local mesenchymal control, the buds form solid branching cords that start to develop a lumen giving rise, by birth, to a network of tubules and alveoli. As the lumen forms, some of the apical cells become structurally polarized and seem to start some secretory activity. The organ develops a stroma containing a large proportion of smooth muscle, whereas the ducts and acini are lined with a layer of flat basal epithelium and a luminal layer of tall columnar secretory epithelium.[4] The basal and luminal epithelial cells are distinguishable on the basis not only of morphology but also functionally and by their expression of different cytokeratin classes (keratins 5 and 14 in basal cells, 8 and 18 in luminal).[5]

Details of prostatic development, in particular molecular details, have been largely established using animal models, in particular the rat and mouse. The availability of tissues from these animals and, more recently, the development of transgenic and gene knock-out models makes them amenable to such studies. Historically, several workers in the field, notably including Dorothy Price, established the basic developmental profile of the rodent prostate.[3,6,7] Rodent prostatic embryogenesis mirrors the processes seen in humans, although the timing reflects the much faster development of these species; for example, an UGS is present in the mouse by embryonic day 16 and in the rat at embryonic day 18 with early prostatic buds being seen a day or so later. Richly illustrated descriptions of the gross[8] and molecular[9] phenotypes of the developing rodent urogenital tract have been published recently that vastly expand the details available in the historic documents. The GenitoUrinary Development Molecular Anatomy Project consortium maintains an updated database of gene expression at its Web site: http://www.gudmap.org.

Growth and development of the prostate begins with formation of prostatic buds from the fetal UGS and are complete at sexual maturity.[10] In the mouse this begins at 17 days gestation,[11,12] at 19 days in the rat,[6] and approximately at 10 weeks in the human fetus.[13,14] The initial event in morphogenesis of the prostate is the outgrowth of solid epithelial buds from the UGS epithelium into the surrounding UGS mesenchyme.[10] The prostatic buds proliferate under the influence of testicular androgens to form solid cords of epithelial cells that grow into the UGS mesenchyme in a particular spatial arrangement to establish the lobar divisions of the prostate.[11,12,14,15] At birth in rodents the prostate is small with a limited number of undeveloped buds; postnatally these cells proliferate, predominantly at the tips,[16] and undergo a process of canalization in a proximal to distal direction (from the urethra toward the tips). Concurrent with this, the epithelial cells differentiate to luminal and basal phenotypes.[17] The prostatic basal cells, at least in rodents, are complex structures with processes that wrap around the ducts; this phenotype is not obvious from traditional histologic sections.[18,19] Concurrent with epithelial differentiation, the UGS mesenchyme proliferates and differentiates into interfasicular fibroblasts and prostatic smooth muscle.[20] Postnatally, under the influence of androgens, the epithelial cells undergo differentiation, including the expression of androgen receptors, and begin to synthesize a variety of lobe- and species-specific secretory products.[21]

In the mouse most prostatic branch points develop before 15 days of age[22] and most of the growth and development of the prostate is complete by 60 days of age.[23] In contrast, the human prostate does not grow significantly between birth and puberty, when growth commences in response to rising androgen levels. The prostate then slowly increases in size over several years. It should be noted that, while androgens drive the development and growth of the prostate, they also play a key role in maintaining a growth-quiescent adult organ. It is noteworthy that young adult males, in whom androgen levels are at their lifetime peak, do not suffer from prostatic enlargement or cancer; rather, these are diseases associated with aging and a decrease in serum androgen titers.

ANATOMY OF THE HUMAN AND RODENT PROSTATE

In 1912, Lowsley[14] used serial sections as anatomic models to describe the lobes of the fetal human prostate to clarify the origin of the middle and posterior lobes as described by earlier investigators.[24] Using tissue from a 3-month gestation fetus, Lowsley identified five separate groups of prostatic ducts originating from the UGS and used the term "lobes" to describe them. These were designated the middle lobe, two lateral, posterior, and ventral lobes. Lowsley described the ventral lobe as being formed by the glands arising from the anterior or ventral wall of the prostatic urethra and consisting of four pairs of epithelial buds. The middle lobe was formed by roughly 12 tubules associated with the posterior urethra and was situated between the bladder and the ejaculatory ducts under the floor of the urethra. The paired left and right lateral tubules, the largest group of tubules, originated from the sides of the urethra and followed the prostatic furrows. The tubules grew laterally and posteriorly, were distal to the ejaculatory ducts, and located on the caudal portion of the urethra, giving rise to the posterior lobe. Although their direction of growth was predominantly toward the bladder, a small number of ducts followed the anterior course of growth as seen in the lateral lobe.

Lowsley's work started a debate over the nomenclature used to describe the prostate anatomy that continued for 70 years or so. In the adult human the lobes that he described are fused and cannot be separated or defined by dissection, giving rise to several different views on the anatomic division of the human prostate.[25–28] The situation is further confused by the fact that, in most other animals, including some other primates, the various prostatic lobes are separable in varying degrees on an anatomic, histologic, and physiologic basis.

The nomenclature that is now most commonly used to describe the structure of the human prostate is that of McNeal.[25] McNeal divided the prostate into three major areas that are histologically distinct and anatomically separate (**Fig. 1**). These areas are the nonglandular fibromuscular stroma that surrounds the organ and the two glandular regions termed peripheral and central zones, which contain a complex yet histologically distinct ductal system. The central zone was described as a wedge of glandular tissue that constitutes most of the base of the prostate and surrounds the ejaculatory ducts. The peripheral zone made up the remainder of the gland. It surrounded most of the central zone and extended caudally to partially

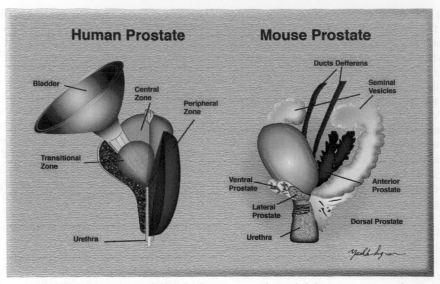

Fig. 1. Structure of human and mouse prostate. (*Left*) Diagram of an adult human prostate showing the urethra and bladder in relation to the three major glandular regions of the prostate as described by McNeal: central zone, peripheral zone, and transitional zone. (*Right*) Diagram depicting the four major prostatic lobes of the mouse prostate, the rat has a similar organization: lateral prostate, dorsal prostate, ventral prostate, and anterior prostate. (*Adapted from* Sugimura Y, Cunha GR, Donjacour AA. Morphogenesis of ductal networks in the mouse prostate. Biol Reprod 1986;34:963; and [left] McNeal JE. Anatomy of the prostate and morphogenesis of BPH. Prog Clin Biol Res 1984;145:27–53.)

surround the distal portion of the urethra. McNeal's classification of the central zone included the middle lobe and part of the posterior lobe described in Lowsley's earlier studies, whereas the peripheral zone included Lowsley's lateral lobes and a portion of the posterior lobe. McNeal also identified an additional, smaller, glandular region that surrounded the prostatitis urethra, referred to as the transition zone.

The peripheral zone ducts exit directly laterally from the posterolateral recesses of the urethral wall. The system consists of small, simple round to oval acinar structures emptying into long narrow ducts surrounded by a stroma of loosely arranged and randomly interwoven muscle bundles. Ducts and acini are lined with simple columnar epithelium. This area is the principal site of prostatitis and carcinoma of the prostate, although not of BPH. The peripheral zone includes the proximal urethral segment of the prostate. This comprises the region of the prostate between the base of the urinary bladder and the verumontanum (the area where the ejaculatory ducts feed into the urethra). The principal feature of this region, which comprises about 5% of the total prostate mass, is the preprostatic sphincter. The sphincter is a cylindrical sleeve of smooth muscle that stretches from the base of the bladder to the verumontanum.

The central zone ducts run predominantly proximally, closely following the ejaculatory ducts.

These ducts and acini are much larger and of irregular contour. The acini are polyhedral in cross-section. The muscular stroma is much more compact than in the peripheral zone. The central zone has a low incidence of disease.

The transitional zone surrounds the urethra between the bladder and the verumontanum. This is a small volume of the prostate, perhaps 5% in the normal organ, but is the principal site of BPH pathogenesis. Nodular expansion of this region of the prostate results in compression of the urethra and the partial bladder outlet obstruction associated with BPH.

Unlike the human, the rodent prostate is not merged into one compact anatomic structure. The rodent prostate is composed of four distinct lobular structures (see **Fig. 1**): (1) anterior lobe (also known as the coagulating gland), (2) dorsal lobe, (3) ventral lobe, and (4) lateral lobe.[16] These lobes exist as pairs on the left and right sides. Because of differences in lobe-specific branching morphogenesis, the final shape of each lobe is distinct.[10]

In rats and mice, the ventral lobes are located immediately below the urinary bladder on the ventral aspect of the urethra. The lateral lobes lie just below the coagulating glands and seminal vesicles, partially overlapping the ventral lobes and dorsally blend with the dorsal lobe.[29,30] The dorsal lobes are found inferior and posterior to the urinary bladder, behind and below the coagulating glands and seminal vesicles. The anterior lobes, or coagulating glands, are directly adjacent to the seminal vesicles.

Lobe/zone homology between the rodent and human prostates has been suggested by various authors. However, the 2001 Bar Harbor Consensus meeting concluded that "there is no existing supporting evidence for a direct relationship between the specific mouse prostate lobes and the specific zones in the human prostate."[31]

ETIOLOGY OF BENIGN PROSTATIC HYPERPLASIA

There are three well-studied conditions that affect the prostate: (1) BPH, (2) prostate cancer, and (3) prostatitis. BPH is a nonmalignant enlargement of the prostate gland and refers to the stromal and glandular epithelial hyperplasia that occurs in the transition zone of the prostate (**Fig. 2**).[32] Clinically, the condition manifests with lower urinary tract symptoms (LUTS) consisting of obstructive (weak urination stream, incomplete bladder emptying, hesitancy) and irritative symptoms (frequency, urgency, nocturia).[33] LUTS can result from a variety of conditions including problems relating to bladder innervation and aging, and the outflow obstruction caused by BPH. LUTS caused by BPH increases with age, and nearly all men develop histologic BPH by 90 years of age.[34] BPH is not generally considered to be a precursor lesion to prostate cancer.

BPH is a common condition linked to aging and the presence of functional testes. McNeal[35–37] proposed the idea that BPH results from a "reawakening" of inductive potential in adult prostatic stroma resulting in focalized formation of new ductal architecture in the transition zone of the prostate (see **Fig. 2**). He described pure stromal nodules and, more commonly, nodules that had been invaded by epithelium to form new glandular architecture. McNeal also made the point that the glands themselves appear normal (**Fig. 3**); it is the overall focal organization that is definitive of BPH (see **Fig. 2**). This is in contrast to the epithelial or stromal hyperplasia seen in many rodent models. These focal nodules adjacent to the urethra give rise to urethral compression and obstruction. One of the central tenets of McNeal's hypothesis was that adult prostatic epithelium should retain an ability to respond to inductive signaling with proliferation and new ductal branching morphogenesis. We, and others, verified this concept for adult rat, mouse, and human prostatic epithelium.[38–40]

Work on canine BPH showed that the condition can be induced with androstanediol and with combinations of androstanediol and estradiol. A combined dose of dihydrotestosterone and estradiol was also found to induce the disease.[41,42] In men, levels of serum testosterone decrease by about 35% between the ages of 21 and 85 against a constant level of estradiol. Thus, there is a change in the androgen/estrogen ratio, which has been suggested to be sufficient to promote the growth of BPH. However, because these changes are not significant until after the first initiation of the disease, their relationship to its induction can be questioned.[43]

McNeal's hypothesis does not address the underlying issue of why "mesenchymal reawakening" may occur or whether there are other etiologic factors in play. Common comorbidities suggest a role for inflammation and possibly metabolic

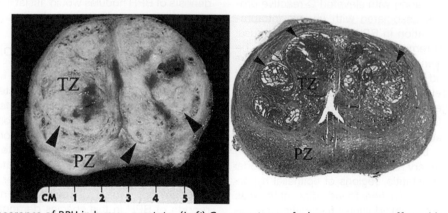

Fig. 2. Appearance of BPH in human prostate. (*Left*) Gross anatomy of a human prostate affected by BPH in the transitional zone. Hyperplastic nodules (*arrowheads*) are clearly visible in the transitional zone (TZ) but not the peripheral zone (PZ) of the gross sample. (*Right*) (H&E) stained wholemount cross-section of a human prostate affected by BPH in the transitional zone. The architectural organization of the glandular structures within the nodules (*arrowheads*) is evident in this low-magnification figure. (*Courtesy of* Scott B. Shappell, MD, PhD, Dallas, TX.)

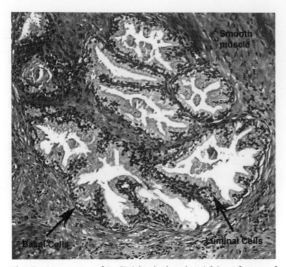

Fig. 3. Structure of individual glands within a focus of BPH. Prostatic glands are composed of columnar luminal epithelial cells and more flattened basal cells surrounded by well-differentiated smooth muscle. Occasional capillaries are seen spaced around the ducts adjacent to the basal epithelium (Hematoxylin and Eosin stain original magnification ×200).

anomalies in the pathogenesis of BPH. Obesity is an epidemic in many developed countries. Low levels of physical activity compound this situation, giving rise to many diseases and patterns of comorbidity including cardiovascular disease, increased insulin resistance, and type II diabetes. Insulin resistance may well be an underlying factor resulting in metabolic syndrome, a condition affecting around 50 million Americans. Metabolic syndrome includes impaired glucose metabolism, elevated weight, altered fat distribution, and hypertension, along with elevated C-reactive protein (which is associated with chronic intraprostatic inflammation in BPH).[44,45] Although causal links to BPH remain unproven, there seems to be a link between metabolic syndrome and LUTS.[46] Diabetes and increased LUTS severity are significantly correlated, even when other covariables, such as age, are factored out.[47]

Obesity is a well-recognized proinflammatory condition, and increased inflammation is closely associated BPH severity, progression, and increased urinary retention.[48,49] In a mouse model of chronic prostatitis, regions of epithelial hyperplasia and dysplasia were found adjacent to areas of inflammation.[50] In addition inflammation, activation of nuclear factor-κB signaling, and subsequent and expression of constitutively active androgen receptor variant 7 have been shown to correlate with BPH progression and prostate volume.[51] Stromal nodules of BPH contain

increased T and B lymphocytes.[52] Elevated levels of inflammatory cells have also been detected in the interstitium and surrounding epithelial glands of human BPH.[53] Infiltration of inflammatory cells in BPH is accompanied by increases in proinflammatory cytokines. Elevated levels of interleukin-2, -8, -17, and interferon-γ have been shown in BPH samples.[54–56] Cytokine expression is seen in early development where the cytokines have direct mitogenic effects on the prostate.[57,58]

The mechanistic basis for the initiation and progression of BPH from asymptomatic to symptomatic remains unclear. Several potential causes have been attributed to the overgrowth of smooth muscle tissue and glandular epithelial tissue in the prostate. These include aging, genetic factors, hormonal changes, and lifestyle.[33,59,60] Although there is still much work to be done to fully understand the basis of BPH progression, such resources as animal models to study BPH are limited and there is a pressing need for new approaches.

BPH was primarily treated surgically for many years. However, in the 1990s this was superseded by the medical approaches that are now front-line therapy. 5α-Reductase inhibitors, such as finasteride and dutasteride, and α-adrenergic blockers, such as doxazosin and tamsulosin, are used to shrink and relax the organ, respectively. The MTOPS study demonstrated that a combination of the α-blocker doxazosin and the 5α-reductase inhibitor finasteride is more effective at reducing LUTS progression than either drug given alone.[48] Although these approaches are effective in many patients, a significant proportion, in the range of 35%, showed progressive disease even in the face of the two-drug combination.[48,49] A detailed understanding of the pathways that lead to the genesis of BPH nodules would assist in the design of better or complementary therapies.

ANIMAL MODELS IN THE STUDY OF BENIGN PROSTATIC HYPERPLASIA

Animal models are necessary for systematic and mechanistic studies of human prostate diseases. The dog and the chimpanzee are the only animals other than humans known to suffer from BPH. As might be expected in a closely related species, the anatomy of the chimpanzee prostate is a close match for the human organ. However, chimpanzees are not a useful experimental model, and reports of BPH in this species demonstrate that, as in humans, the disease is sporadic and associated with aging.[61] Historically several studies were performed on spontaneously arising BPH in the canine prostate. Canine BPH, like its human counterpart, arises with increasing frequency with age and requires functional testes. The diseases differ, in that human BPH is strongly focal with distinct nodules of hyperplasia within the gland, whereas the canine disease is diffuse, occurring throughout the gland.[42,62] In the dog, there is therefore a general expansion of the gland, which is less anatomically fixed than in humans, resulting in compression of the rectum, producing constipation as a symptom as opposed to the urinary retention found in humans. Practical considerations, notably that the disease occurs in older animals (generally >8 years) and the costs associated with maintaining colonies of large mammals, have severely limited work in this model.

BPH in humans has several common components; the essential element is the focal nodular growth that usually occurs close to the urethra. There is also commonly inflammation and the activation of associated transcription factors, such as nuclear factor-κB, and upregulation of the androgen receptor and constitutively active variants. This process is associated with compression of the urethra and LUTS caused by partial bladder outlet obstruction. The anatomy of the rodent prostate largely precludes the recapitulation of all of these characteristics in a single model. For this reason it is important to assess which particular aspects of the human disease are present in any given model. Most of the models that are available develop some form of hyperplasia, either of the epithelium, stroma, or both; however, the glandular structures are generally histologically abnormal, and appropriate caution must be exercised in interpreting the data. Focalized glandular expansion with normal-appearing new glands, as seen in human BPH nodules, is not evident in most animal models. For these reasons, most of these should not be considered models of BPH, but, rather, of whichever processes of the disease they most accurately reflect.

Manipulating the hormonal environment has been used in rats to induce prostate cancer.[63] Similar manipulations can also be applied to induce bladder outflow obstruction and inflammation.[64] Applying such a regimen to mice to mimic the changes in the testosterone/estrogen ratio seen in the aging human male results in bladder outflow obstruction and urination patterns that in some ways mirror human LUTS.[65] In this model there are increases in glandular ducts surrounding the proximal urethra with the potential to compress this structure and give rise to a partial bladder outlet obstruction.

Several transgenic, knock-out and knock-in mouse models have been described with various prostatic phenotypes. These include a prostate-specific 15-LOX-2 transgenic mouse generated using the ARR2PB promoter allowing for targeted expression of 15-LOX-2 or 15-LOX-2sv-b, a splice variant lacking arachidonic acid-metabolizing activity. These manipulations resulted in age-dependent increases in prostatic wet weight with predominantly epithelial hyperplasia.[66] A conditional knockout of PPARγ in the mouse prostate also resulted in increases in prostate size with epithelial hyperplasia that progressed to prostatic intraepithelial neoplasia and occasional cancer.[67] This observation makes the point that epithelial hyperplasia in the mouse might be an early premalignant change, clearly differentiating it from human BPH.

Nonobese diabetic mice represent a model of immune dysregulation and type I diabetes. First reported in 1980, these mice exhibit spontaneous development of autoimmune insulin-dependent diabetes mellitus.[68] These mice are important because the autoimmune response is not fully penetrant; as a result, subgroups of mice exhibit diabetes, with or without prostatic inflammation. This allows for independent assessment of the effects of these two human BPH-relevant variables. Histochemical analysis reveals a reduction of the epithelium and increased stroma. As a result, muscular and collagen hypertrophy in the prostatic gland when inflammation occurs.[69] In noninflamed but nonobese diabetic/severe combined immune deficiency mice, a strong epithelial hyperplastic phenotype in the anterior and ventral prostate has been noted.[70]

SUMMARY

Many researchers have studied the embryology, development, and anatomy of the human prostate. Debates over the nomenclature to describe the gland have been settled and standardized nomenclature exists. BPH is a complex disease that probably has multiple causes often occurring in patients with complex comorbidities, prominently including obesity and diabetes.

Animal models have proven to be useful in understanding the underlying mechanisms of many human diseases. However, the structure of the human and rodent prostates is very different. Extrapolation of data between species requires an understanding of these differences and of the limitations of specific models.

REFERENCES

1. Saunders JBdeCM, O'Malley CD. The illustrations from the works of Andreas Vesalius of Brussels: with annotations and translations, a discussion of the plates and their background, authorship and

influence, and a biographical sketch of Vesalius. Cleveland (OH): World Publishing Company; 1950.

2. Geller J. Pathogenesis and medical treatment of benign prostatic hyperplasia. Prostate Suppl 1989; 2:95–104.

3. Price D, Williams-Ashman H. The accessory reproductive glands of mammals. In: Young W, editor. Sex and internal secretions, vol. 1, 3rd edition. Baltimore (MD): Williams and Wilkins; 1961. p. 366–448.

4. Shapiro E, Hartanto V, Lepor H. Quantifying the smooth muscle content of the prostate using double-immunoenzymatic staining and color assisted image analysis. J Urol 1992;147:1167–70.

5. Josso N. Physiology of sex differentiation. In: Josso N, editor. The Intersex Child, Pediatric and Adolescent Endocrinology, vol. 8. Basel (Switzerland): Karger; 1981. p. 1–13.

6. Price D. Normal development of the prostate and seminal vesicles of the rat with a study of experimental postnatal modifications. Am J Anat 1936;60(1):79–127.

7. Price D. Comparative aspects of development and structure in the prostate. Natl Cancer Inst Monogr 1963;12:1–27.

8. Staack A, Donjacour AA, Brody J, et al. Mouse urogenital development: a practical approach. Differentiation 2003;71(7):402–13.

9. Georgas KM, Armstrong J, Keast JR, et al. An illustrated anatomical ontology of the developing mouse lower urogenital tract. Development 2015;142(10): 1893–908.

10. Marker PC, Donjacour AA, Dahiya R, et al. Hormonal, cellular, and molecular control of prostatic development. Dev Biol 2003;253(2):165–74.

11. Cunha GR, Donjacour AA, Cooke PS, et al. The endocrinology and developmental biology of the prostate. Endocr Rev 1987;8(3):338–62.

12. Timms BG, Mohs TJ, Didio LJ. Ductal budding and branching patterns in the developing prostate. J Urol 1994;151(5):1427–32.

13. Kellokumpu-Lehtinen P, Santti R, Pelliniemi LJ. Correlation of early cytodifferentiation of the human fetal prostate and Leydig cells. Anat Rec 1980; 196(3):263–73.

14. Lowsley OS. The development of the human prostate gland with reference to the development of other structures at the neck of the urinary bladder. Am J Anat 1912;13(3):299–349.

15. Kellokumpu-Lehtinen P. Development of sexual dimorphism in human urogenital sinus complex. Biol Neonate 1985;48(3):157–67.

16. Sugimura Y, Cunha GR, Donjacour AA, et al. Whole-mount autoradiography study of DNA synthetic activity during postnatal development and androgen-induced regeneration in the mouse prostate. Biol Reprod 1986;34(5):985–95.

17. Hayward SW, Baskin LS, Haughney PC, et al. Epithelial development in the rat ventral prostate, anterior prostate and seminal vesicle. Acta Anat (Basel) 1996;155:81–93.

18. Hayward SW, Brody JR, Cunha GR. An edgewise look at basal cells: three-dimensional views of the rat prostate, mammary gland and salivary gland. Differentiation 1996;60:219–27.

19. Soeffing WJ, Timms BG. Localization of androgen receptor and cell-specific cytokeratins in basal cells of rat ventral prostate. J Androl 1995;16(3):197–208.

20. Hayward SW, Baskin LS, Haughney PC, et al. Stromal development in the ventral prostate, anterior prostate and seminal vesicle of the rat. Acta Anat (Basel) 1996;155(2):94–103.

21. Timms BG. Prostate development: a historical perspective. Differentiation 2008;76(6):565–77.

22. Sugimura Y, Cunha GR, Donjacour AA. Morphogenesis of ductal networks in the mouse prostate. Biol Reprod 1986;34:961–71.

23. Donjacour AA, Cunha GR. The effect of androgen deprivation on branching morphogenesis in the mouse prostate. Dev Biol 1988;128(1):1–14.

24. Evatt EJ. A contribution to the development of the prostate in man. J Anat Physiol 1909;43(Pt 4): 314–21.

25. McNeal JE. Anatomy of the prostate and morphogenesis of BPH. Prog Clin Biol Res 1984;145:27–53.

26. Franks LM. Benign nodular hyperplasia of the prostate: a review. Ann R Coll Surg Engl 1954;14:92–106.

27. Hutch JA, Rambo ON. A study of the anatomy of the prostate, prostatic urethra and the urinary sphincter system. J Urol 1970;105:443–52.

28. Tissell LE, Salander H. Anatomy of the human prostate and its three paired lobes. Prog Clin Biol Res 1984;145:55–66.

29. Hayashi N, Sugimura Y, Kawamura J, et al. Morphological and functional heterogeneity in the rat prostatic gland. Biol Reprod 1991;45(2):308–21.

30. Roy-Burman P, Wu H, Powell WC, et al. Genetically defined mouse models that mimic natural aspects of human prostate cancer development. Endocr Relat Cancer 2004;11(2):225–54.

31. Shappell SB, Thomas GV, Roberts RL, et al. Prostate pathology of genetically engineered mice: definitions and classification. The consensus report from the Bar Harbor meeting of the mouse models of Human Cancer Consortium Prostate Pathology Committee. Cancer Res 2004;64(6):2270–305.

32. Dhingra N, Bhagwat D. Benign prostatic hyperplasia: an overview of existing treatment. Indian J Pharmacol 2011;43(1):6–12.

33. Miller J, Tarter TH. Combination therapy with dutasteride and tamsulosin for the treatment of symptomatic enlarged prostate. Clin Interv Aging 2009;4: 251–8.

34. Berry SJ, Coffey DS, Walsh PC, et al. The development of human benign prostatic hyperplasia with age. J Urol 1984;132(3):474–9.

35. McNeal JE. The prostate gland: morphology and pathobiology. Monogr Urol 1988;4:3–37.

36. McNeal JE. Origin and evolution of benign prostatic enlargement. Invest Urol 1978;15(4):340–5.

37. McNeal JE. Morphology and biology of benign prostatic hyperplasia. In: Bruchovsky N, Chapdellaine A, Neumann F, editors. Regulation of androgen action. Berlin: Congressdruck R. Bruckner; 1985. p. 191–7.

38. Norman JT, Cunha GR, Sugimura Y. The induction of new ductal growth in adult prostatic epithelium in response to an embryonic prostatic inductor. Prostate 1986;8:209–20.

39. Hayashi N, Cunha GR, Parker M. Permissive and instructive induction of adult rodent prostatic epithelium by heterotypic urogenital sinus mesenchyme. Epithelial Cell Biol 1993;2(2):66–78.

40. Hayward SW, Haughney PC, Rosen MA, et al. Interactions between adult human prostatic epithelium and rat urogenital sinus mesenchyme in a tissue recombination model. Differentiation 1998;63(3):131–40.

41. Walsh PC, Wilson JD. The induction of prostatic hypertrophy in the dog with androstanediol. J Clin Invest 1976;57:1093–7.

42. DeKlerk DP, Coffey DS, Ewing LL, et al. Comparison of spontaneous and experimentally induced canine prostatic hyperplasia. J Clin Invest 1979;64(3):842–9.

43. Wilson JD. The pathogenesis of benign prostatic hyperplasia. Am J Med 1980;68:745–56.

44. Kasturi S, Russell S, McVary KT. Metabolic syndrome and lower urinary tract symptoms secondary to benign prostatic hyperplasia. Curr Urol Rep 2006;7(4):288–92.

45. Rohrmann S, De Marzo AM, Smit E, et al. Serum C-reactive protein concentration and lower urinary tract symptoms in older men in the Third National Health and Nutrition Examination Survey (NHANES III). Prostate 2005;62(1):27–33.

46. Hammarsten J, Hogstedt B. Clinical, haemodynamic, anthropometric, metabolic and insulin profile of men with high-stage and high-grade clinical prostate cancer. Blood Press 2004;13(1):47–55.

47. Michel MC, Mehlburger L, Schumacher H, et al. Effect of diabetes on lower urinary tract symptoms in patients with benign prostatic hyperplasia. J Urol 2000;163(6):1725–9.

48. McConnell JD, Roehrborn CG, Bautista OM, et al. The long-term effect of doxazosin, finasteride, and combination therapy on the clinical progression of benign prostatic hyperplasia. N Engl J Med 2003;349(25):2387–98.

49. McVary KT. A review of combination therapy in patients with benign prostatic hyperplasia. Clin Ther 2007;29(3):387–98.

50. Elkahwaji JE, Zhong W, Hopkins WJ, et al. Chronic bacterial infection and inflammation incite reactive hyperplasia in a mouse model of chronic prostatitis. Prostate 2007;67(1):14–21.

51. Austin DC, Strand DW, Love HL, et al. NF-kappaB and androgen receptor variant expression correlate with human BPH progression. Prostate 2015;76(5):491–511.

52. Bierhoff E, Vogel J, Benz M, et al. Stromal nodules in benign prostatic hyperplasia. Eur Urol 1996;29(3):345–54.

53. Theyer G, Kramer G, Assmann I, et al. Phenotypic characterization of infiltrating leukocytes in benign prostatic hyperplasia. Lab Invest 1992;66(1):96–107.

54. Kramer G, Steiner GE, Handisurya A, et al. Increased expression of lymphocyte-derived cytokines in benign hyperplastic prostate tissue, identification of the producing cell types, and effect of differentially expressed cytokines on stromal cell proliferation. Prostate 2002;52(1):43–58.

55. Steiner GE, Stix U, Handisurya A, et al. Cytokine expression pattern in benign prostatic hyperplasia infiltrating T cells and impact of lymphocytic infiltration on cytokine mRNA profile in prostatic tissue. Lab Invest 2003;83(8):1131–46.

56. Giri D, Ittmann M. Interleukin-8 is a paracrine inducer of fibroblast growth factor 2, a stromal and epithelial growth factor in benign prostatic hyperplasia. Am J Pathol 2001;159(1):139–47.

57. Jerde TJ, Bushman W. IL-1 induces IGF-dependent epithelial proliferation in prostate development and reactive hyperplasia. Sci Signal 2009;2(86):ra49.

58. Wang L, Zoetemelk M, Chitteti BR, et al. Expansion of prostate epithelial progenitor cells after inflammation of the mouse prostate. Am J Physiol Renal Physiol 2015;308(12):F1421–30.

59. Culig Z, Hobisch A, Cronauer MV, et al. Regulation of prostatic growth and function by peptide growth factors. Prostate 1996;28(6):392–405.

60. Jenkins EP, Andersson S, Imperato-McGinley J, et al. Genetic and pharmacological evidence for more than one human steroid 5 alpha-reductase. J Clin Invest 1992;89(1):293–300.

61. Steiner MS, Couch RC, Raghow S, et al. The chimpanzee as a model of human benign prostatic hyperplasia. J Urol 1999;162(4):1454–61.

62. Berry SJ, Strandberg JD, Saunders WJ, et al. Development of canine benign prostatic hyperplasia with age. Prostate 1986;9(4):363–73.

63. Noble RL. The development of prostatic adenocarcinoma in Nb rats following prolonged sex hormone administration. Cancer Res 1977;37(6):1929–33.

64. Bernoulli J, Yatkin E, Konkol Y, et al. Prostatic inflammation and obstructive voiding in the adult Noble rat: impact of the testosterone to estradiol ratio in serum. Prostate 2008;68(12):1296–306.

65. Nicholson TM, Ricke EA, Marker PC, et al. Testosterone and 17beta-estradiol induce glandular prostatic growth, bladder outlet obstruction, and voiding dysfunction in male mice. Endocrinology 2012;153(11):5556–65.

66. Suraneni MV, Schneider-Broussard R, Moore JR, et al. Transgenic expression of 15-lipoxygenase 2 (15-LOX2) in mouse prostate leads to hyperplasia and cell senescence. Oncogene 2010;29(30): 4261–75.

67. Jiang M, Fernandez S, Jerome WG, et al. Disruption of PPARgamma signaling results in mouse prostatic intraepithelial neoplasia involving active autophagy. Cell Death Differ 2010;17(3):469–81.

68. Makino S, Kunimoto K, Muraoka Y, et al. Breeding of a non-obese, diabetic strain of mice. Jikken Dobutsu 1980;29(1):1–13.

69. Ribeiro DL, Caldeira EJ, Candido EM, et al. Prostatic stromal microenvironment and experimental diabetes. Eur J Histochem 2006;50(1):51–60.

70. Jiang M, Strand DW, Franco OE, et al. PPARgamma: a molecular link between systemic metabolic disease and benign prostate hyperplasia. Differentiation 2011;82(4–5):220–36.

The Epidemiology of Benign Prostatic Hyperplasia Associated with Lower Urinary Tract Symptoms
Prevalence and Incident Rates

Kathryn Brigham Egan, PhD, MPH[a,b]

KEYWORDS

- Benign prostatic hyperplasia • Lower urinary tract symptoms • Aging • Urology • Prostate disease
- Incidence • Prevalence

KEY POINTS

- Prevalence and incidence rates for benign prostatic hyperplasia and lower urinary tract symptoms (BPH/LUTS) have not previously been summarized in the literature by age group, symptom severity, and/or race/ethnicity.
- BPH/LUTS prevalence rates ranged from 50% to 75% among men 50 years of age and older to 80% among men 70 years of age and older. Overall incidence rates ranged from 8.5 to 41 cases/1000 person–years.
- BPH/LUTS epidemiologic estimates generally increased with increasing age. Unmeasured cultural, psychosocial, economic, and/or medical reporting differences may contribute to reported differences by age and symptom severity.

INTRODUCTION

Benign prostatic hyperplasia (BPH) is a prevalent condition in aging men that represents a substantial disease burden. It can be associated with various other health outcomes that can have significant negative impacts on quality of life. Many men with BPH will never see a doctor, nor will they need treatment for the condition.[1] BPH becomes a clinical entity when lower urinary tract symptoms (LUTS) associated with it are bothersome enough for a patient to seek medical care. LUTS is the preferred terminology to describe symptoms potentially caused by multiple pathologic conditions, including bladder storage symptoms and voiding difficulties such as increased urgency, frequent urination, weak urinary stream, and urine leakage.[2,3] BPH/LUTS, or benign prostatic hyperplasia associated with lower urinary tract symptoms, affects more than 20% of American men aged 30 to 79 years,[3] or roughly 15 million men. This prevalence appears to increase with increasing age, as approximately 80% of men are affected by BPH/LUTS by 70 years of age.[4] Most men, if living long enough, will develop some histologic features consistent with BPH in their lifetime.[1]

To date, no reviews have focused on the prevalence and incidence of BPH/LUTS overall or by disease severity, patient age, and/or race/ethnicity. The primary aim of this article is to assess the full body of published literature in regard to BPH/LUTS estimates as well as to

Disclosure Statement: The author has no relevant financial information to disclose.
a Yale University, 2 Whalley Ave, New Haven, CT 06520, USA; b New England Research Institutes Inc., 480 Pleasant Street, Watertown, MA 02472, USA
E-mail address: Katie.Brigham@gmail.com

Urol Clin N Am 43 (2016) 289–297
http://dx.doi.org/10.1016/j.ucl.2016.04.001

determine if the differences reported by disease severity, age, and race/ethnicity are consistent between studies and/or comparable. The variation in disease definition and assessment used for studies of BPH/LUTS prevalence and incidence rates may make comparing reported rates between studies complicated and sometimes, impossible.

DISEASE DESCRIPTION/TERMINOLOGY
Benign Prostatic Hyperplasia

Clinical BPH is a histologic diagnosis of a progressive enlargement of the prostate gland resulting from nonmalignant proliferation of smooth muscle and epithelial prostate cells.[5] BPH disease progression can lead to growth in the transition zone of the prostate gland, called benign prostatic enlargement (BPE), which results from proliferation of fibroblasts and epithelial glandular elements near the urethra.[6,7] Men with clinical BPH typically have prostate volumes of at least 20 mL.[8]

Lower Urinary Tract Symptoms

Fifty percent of men with BPH develop BPE, which can contribute to LUTS that include a broad range of symptoms and etiologies.[8] Clinical diagnosis of BPH/LUTS is a multistep process, with the definition used in the literature and in clinical studies varying widely. LUTS are presently divided into either bladder storage symptoms, such as daytime urinary frequency, urgency, and nocturia; or emptying and voiding difficulties, such as straining, starting the stream of urine, intermittent stream, and incomplete emptying. Not all men with storage or voiding difficulties will be bothered by these symptoms and so may not seek medical attention.[1] However, early BPH/LUTS detection and appropriate management may improve quality of life outcomes and help to prevent more severe disease consequences. Despite this, men generally do not seek BPH treatment until the corresponding LUTS significantly reduce their quality of life.[9]

One way to assess BPH/LUTS severity in men is by using the validated, self-administered International Prostate Symptom Score (IPSS). The IPSS is the present international standard evaluating 7 of the most common storage and voiding LUTS. It is also known as the American Urologic Symptom Index (AUA-SI). Severity is traditionally classified as

No more than 7 points = none or mild
8 to 20 points = moderate
20 to 35 points = severe

A strong correlation between symptom severity and frequency as measured by IPSS and other measures, such as the BPH Impact Index and the Symptom Problem Index, have been documented.[10] IPSS can be used to diagnose LUTS in conjunction with a transrectal ultrasound of the prostate, a measurement of maximal urinary flow rate (Q_{max}) and/or a measurement of postvoid residual volume assessed by ultrasound, serum prostate-specific antigen levels, or urinalysis.[8,11,12]

RISK FACTORS AND COMORBIDITIES

Medical and lifestyle predictors of BPH/LUTS have been primarily studied despite the high disease burden that should prompt researchers to assess population-level BPH/LUTS sociodemographic and environmental risk factors.

Known risk factors associated with BPH/LUTS[12–16] include

- Age
- Sedentary lifestyle
- Lack of exercise
- Smoking
- Excessive alcohol consumption
- Hypertension
- Type II diabetes
- Depression
- Cardiovascular disease
- Hyperlipidemia
- Central obesity/waist circumference
- Hypogonadism
- Prostate disorder
- Inflammation
- Genetic predisposition

Risk factors have been shown to increase the risk of BPH/LUTS[16,17] include

- Age
- Diabetes
- Hypertension
- Obesity
- Hypogonadism

Risk factors shown to decrease the risk of BPH/LUTS[16] include

- Increased physical activity
- Moderate or decreased alcohol intake
- Increased vegetable consumption

The comorbidities often associated with BPH/LUTS[12,13,18,19] include

- Erectile dysfunction
- Ejaculatory dysfunction
- Hypertension

- High cholesterol
- Digestive tract disorder
- Arthritis
- Heart disease/heart failure
- Diabetes
- Depression/anxiety/sleep disorder
- Allergies/cold/influenza/congestion
- General pain/inflammation

PREVALENCE/INCIDENCE

Disentangling BPH, LUTS, and BPH/LUTS prevalence and incidence rates reported in the literature is difficult due to the varying disease definitions and assessment methods used between studies.[20] Because of these differences in disease definitions and reporting methods such as self-report qualitative and/or quantitative symptoms or diagnoses versus medical record reviews performed by trained medical professionals, BPH, LUTS, and BPH/LUTS estimates in the literature should be interpreted with caution, as inappropriately comparing or combining estimates of the different conditions could lead to potentially inaccurate conclusions.

Prevalence

Overall and by age

An estimated 15 million men in the United States over the age of 30 years are affected by BPH/LUTS.[21] Large variations in existing prevalence rates are reported due to differences in BPH/LUTS definitions, assessment methods, and geographic regions. As presented in **Fig. 1**,

BPH/LUTS prevalence estimates also vary by age.[15,22–26] Among men over the age of 50 years, 50% to 75% experience BPH/LUTS.[22,27,28] For the majority of these men, without treatment, voiding and storage symptoms will significantly worsen with increasing age and time.[21] Among men over the age of 70 years, 80% on average are impacted by BPH/LUTS.

As presented in **Fig. 1**, the BPH/LUTS prevalence estimates reported in the literature vary. Despite this variation, the histologic prevalence of BPH/LUTS typically increased with increasing age in each study as androgens and aging are necessary for the development of BPH/LUTS.[1,29] Prostate enlargement, peak flow rate, and LUTS have all been shown to be age-dependent conditions and are conditions that play a substantial role in BPH/LUTS development among aging men.[30] Urinary symptoms of urgency, nocturia, weak stream, intermittency, and incomplete emptying are the most strongly correlated with age,[31] and prevalence estimates rise to as high as 88% to 90% by 81 years of age or greater.[4,22,28,31,32]

By disease severity

BPH/LUTS severity varies within each reported overall prevalence rate. The BPH Registry and Patient Survey, a prospective observational disease registry documenting BPH/LUTS practices and patient outcomes among 6909 men in the United States, reported that 33% of men had mild LUTS; 52% of men had moderate LUTS, and 15% of men had severe LUTS.[13] The

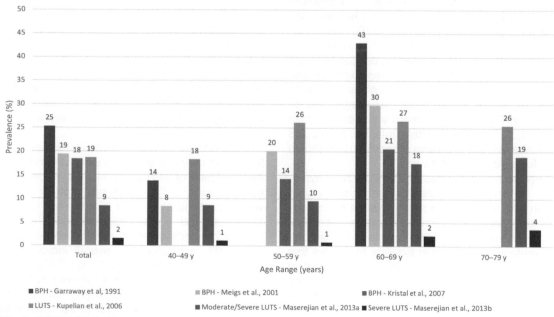

Fig. 1. BPH/LUTS prevalence estimates among men 40 to 80 years of age.

average IPSS at baseline was 11.6 (range 0–35).[13] Another study based in the United States reported that 72.3% of men sometimes have LUTS, and 47.9% often have LUTS when LUTS were self-reported on a 5-point Likert scale.[19] Bosch and colleagues[33] reported moderate LUTS among 24% and severe LUTS among 6% of men in a community-based population survey of men between the ages of 55 and 74 years. In France, when LUTS were assessed via IPSS, 67% of men scored 1≤IPSS less than 8 (mild), 13% scored 8≤IPSS less than 19 (moderate), and 1.2% scored 20≤IPSS (severe).[34] Another cross-sectional study supported these results, with a reported prevalence of mild symptoms among all symptomatic men equal to 75%, moderate symptoms equal to 21%, and severe symptoms equal to 4%.[35] Among only men aged 40 to 49 years, these prevalence estimates for mild, moderate, and severe symptoms were 89%, 9%, and 2%, respectively. This increased to 55% with mild, 37% with moderate, and 8% with severe LUTS among men over the age of 70 years.[35]

The reported differences in BPH/LUTS severity could be caused by differences in disease etiology that are currently poorly understood. Approximately 10% of men ≤30 years old, 20% of men 30 to 40 years old, 50% to 60% of men 40 to 60 years old, and greater than 80% of men 80 or more years old have enlarged prostates.[36] Prostate volume generally increases with age, although rates vary at the individual level, and prostate volume is associated with BPH/LUTS.[36] Men with significant prostate enlargement (>50 cm³) are 3.5 times more likely to have age-adjusted moderate-to-severe LUTS than men without prostate enlargement.[37] However, in another study[33] only a weak correlation between IPSS, peak flow, and postvoid residual urine volumes and prostate volume was observed due to the simple fact that most men, regardless of LUTS severity, have prostate volumes less than 50 mL.[38,39] Looking further into the BPH/LUTS disease etiology is an area of research that should be focused on in the future.

Prevalence estimates for BPH/LUTS by symptom severity should also be further studied, as men with more severe symptoms are more likely to seek treatment, which may bias estimates, especially in studies utilizing convenience samples of urology patients. This extends to studies that utilize medical record reviews, as most tend to include only men with moderate-to-severe symptoms as those are the men seeking treatment and, therefore, receiving BPH/LUTS diagnoses for data extraction.

By race/ethnicity

BPH/LUTS prevalence estimates are infrequently reported by race/ethnicity. Many studies included in this article have primarily racially homogenous populations and are, therefore, unable to draw conclusions on racial or ethnic differences in disease prevalence. However, there are a select few published articles of heterogeneous populations that are able to assess this difference, and these studies tend to indicate that the prevalence of BPH/LUTS may vary by race/ethnicity. The Prostate Cancer Prevention Trial reported the highest prevalence of BPH to be among Hispanic men, followed by black, white, and Asian men.[15] This mirrored the results of the California Men's Health Study and the Research Program in Genes, Environment and Health, which reported the highest prevalence of LUTS among Hispanic men, followed by black, white, and Asian men.[40] Additionally, black men had an estimated moderate-to-severe LUTS prevalence of 39.6% in the Flint Men's Health Study.[41] Other studies reported that Japanese, Chinese, and Indian men have significantly lower prostate volumes than Australian or American men, which could contribute to BPH/LUTS prevalence differences.[42,43] Additionally, the Third National Health and Nutrition Examination Survey (NHANES) reported some LUTS prevalence estimates by race/ethnicity. However, these NHANES estimates did not include the full spectrum of urinary symptoms as assessed by IPSS and are, therefore, unfortunately, not comparable to other BPH/LUTS race/ethnicity estimates presented here.[44]

Incidence

Overall

Fig. 2 shows the overall incidence rates reported by 4 BPH/LUTS longitudinal cohort studies: The Prostate Cancer Prevention Trial, The Olmstead County study, The Health Professionals Follow-up Study, and a database review in the Netherlands.[15,25,45,46]

The Prostate Cancer Prevention Trial included 5667 men over the age of 55 years and reported the incidence of BPH to be 34.4 cases per 1000 person–years.[15] The Olmstead County study, which identified men living in Olmstead County, Minnesota, with a new clinical diagnosis of BPH verified by medical record review between 1987 and 1997, estimated the overall incidence of BPH to be 8.54 cases per 1000 men.[25] The Health Professionals Follow-up Study followed 9628 men with moderate-to-severe LUTS (8≤IPSS<14) and 2557 men with severe LUTS (IPSS ≥20) from LUTS onset for an average of 12.7 years to assess

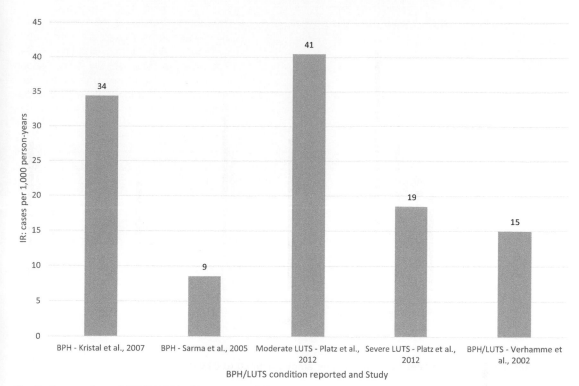

Fig. 2. Comparsion of BPH/LUTS incidence rates (IR).

LUTS incidence and progression rates. Incidence rates of moderate and severe LUTS were 41 and 19 cases per 1000 person–years, respectively.[46] Verhamme and colleagues[45] utilized a longitudinal observational database in the Netherlands to assess incidence rates of BPH/LUTS among men over the age of 45 years who had at least 6 months of patient follow-up and reported the incidence of BPH/LUTS to be 15 cases per 1000 person–years of follow-up.

By age and disease severity

As with prevalence rates, reported incidence rates differ by age at disease onset, duration of follow-up, patient age at follow-up, and study design. Additionally, disease severity and how it is measured impact reported incidence rates, as they vary not only by age, but also by symptom severity and patient tolerance of those symptoms.

The 4 studies with overall estimates mentioned previously also reported incidence rates by age and/or severity. The increasing incidence of BPH/LUTS by age group is presented in **Fig. 3**.[15,25,45,46]

The Prostate Cancer Prevention Trial reported that for every 1 year increase in patient age, the incidence of BPH increased by 4%.[15] This corresponds to reports that an estimated 45% of urinary symptom-free men over the age of 45 will develop BPH/LUTS before the age of 75.[45] The Health Professionals Follow-up Study reported increases in both moderate and severe LUTS incidence rates with increasing patient age.[46] Verhamme and colleagues[45] reported the incidence of BPH to linearly increase by an average of 6.15 cases per 1000 man–years for every 5-year increase in age increment between 45 and 79 years of age. This increase was from 3 cases per 1000 man–years age 45 to 49 to 38 cases per 1000 man–years at age 75 to 79 years.[45] Interestingly, the linear increase in incidence rates stopped after 80 years of age, and this increase has been similarly documented in other BPH symptom studies.[47,48] After age 80 years, any further increase may be attenuated by a healthy survivor effect or by underreporting of LUTS among elderly men who may or may not report symptoms in a similar manner as younger men.

By race/ethnicity

Incidence rates, for the same reasons as prevalence rates, are also seldom presented in the literature for BPH/LUTS. The California Men's Health Study and the Research Program in Genes, Environment and Health reported Asian men to have a lower risk of moderate-to-severe LUTS than white men and that LUTS incidence increases with each increasing baseline age for all race/ethnic groups (32%–56%).[40]

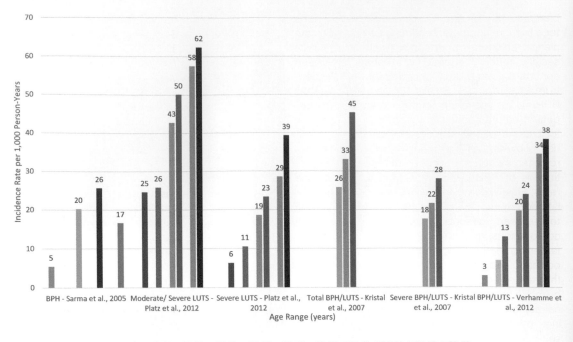

Fig. 3. BPH/LUTS incidence rates by study and age among men 40 to 80 years old.

DISCUSSION

Benign Prostatic Hyperplasia and Lower Urinary Tract Symptoms Estimates: Comparison

The relationship between BPH, LUTS, bladder outlet obstruction, and benign prostatic enlargement is complex. This complexity can lead to problems with epidemiologic definitions between studies.

There are several factors that complicate BPH/LUTS prevalence and incidence rate comparisons. First, there is an insufficient consensus on the epidemiologic definition of BPH, LUTS, and BPH/LUTS. Different studies often calculate prevalence and incidence using different disease definitions and assessment methods. Also, even if similar incidence and prevalence definitions are used, they are often stratified using varying analysis-dependent symptom cut-offs.[20] This variation in disease definition makes comparisons difficult to interpret, and conclusions drawn should be interpreted with caution. Therefore, epidemiologic studies reporting on the prevalence and incidence of disease need to include data on specific symptoms, disease definition, prostate size, and urinary flow for all study participants.[49–51] Second, the evaluation of a few self-report urinary symptoms in lieu of reporting on all LUTS, as assessed by a validated scale such as the IPSS, provides insufficient data for comparison between studies.

This incomplete assessment of LUTS may or may not be related to BPH prevalence in the assessed population and therefore is not useful for overall, age-dependent, or severity-dependent comparisons between studies. Third, cultural, psychosocial, and economic factors may play an influential role in the reported BPH/LUTS prevalence rates, as these factors may influence access to medical care, symptom reporting, interactions with health care providers, and help-seeking behaviors.[52] Fourth, the timing of self-report questionnaires should be considered when designing either cross-sectional or longitudinal urologic studies, as BPH/LUTS prevalence and incidence rates vary by baseline age, follow-up age, and symptom severity. Recall periods often differed among the studies reviewed, and, as BPH/LUTS vary over time, recall bias may contribute to fluctuations in rates, as men may report symptoms differently depending on their age at assessment. Fifth, the likelihood of responder bias being present in the reported estimates from cohorts of men seeking medical attention should be noted, as men with symptoms may be more likely to respond to surveys in comparison to men with no symptoms. Cohorts of patients seeking medical attention can also have socioeconomic factor bias such as access to health care which can skew results. The type of cohort used for analysis varied widely by study. Again, this bias may vary by age. Community-based cohorts tend to more accurately estimate BPH/LUTS prevalence rates than cohorts of self-selected patients seeking medical attention, as community-based cohorts are more likely to represent the full spectrum of symptoms. Sixth, studies should assess BPH/LUTS treatment sought by each individual patient before administering study questionnaires for cross-sectional surveys and/or after longitudinal follow-up, as treatment could impact men's reported symptom severity and result in underestimates of BPH/LUTS prevalence and incidence rates. Finally, sample selection and survey administration methods varied across studies and need to be clearly described in reports when making comparisons, as demographic and environmental factors of included populations may impact reported outcomes. Because of the sensitivity of the requested information, responses may differ by mode of survey administration: postal questionnaires, in-person or telephone interviews, screenings by medical professionals, and/or in-person self-administer questionnaires.

CLINICAL CORRELATION

Worldwide, populations are aging. This correlates to an increase in the number of older men and an increase in life expectancy. As BPH/LUTS is an age-related disease that increases in prevalence and incidence as men get older, appropriate management and use of resources for BPH/LUTS, and other age-related conditions, is a major challenge for the health care system. Recently, there has been a shift from surgical procedures to medical therapy for BPH/LUTS treatment. This is thought to be a result of men with LUTS reporting significant decreases in their quality of life.[13] This shift in treatment type, the increase in the disease burden as more treatment is sought, and a decrease in the number of practicing urologists per capita have created a need to better understand BPH/LUTS physician practices and patient outcomes.

BPH/LUTS outcomes may be additionally confounded by environmental, socioeconomic and/or demographic factors of which clinicians should be aware. Despite the high BPH/LUTS disease burden, sociographic and environmental factors have been insufficiently studied in favor of medical and lifestyle predictors. In one of the few studies to date of sociodemographic factors, the Boston Area Community Health (BACH) study reported that the differences in incidence were found to be almost wholly attributable to the mediating effects of education and income, rather than ethnic or racial differences among men.[26]

However, this influence has rarely been studied elsewhere. Also, BACH did not assess the degree of urbanization within their cohort and urbanization's potential effects on recognition or management of LUTS. Men in urbanized settings with increased access to advanced medical care may be more likely to report LUTS or seek treatment for BPH/LUTS, but this association needs to be further investigated.

SUMMARY

The number of men diagnosed with BPH/LUTS in the last decade has been increasing over time. Prostate enlargement, specifically BPH, has been shown to be associated with the symptomatic progression of LUTS. Numerous cross-sectional and longitudinal studies have provided data on BPH, LUTS, and BPH/LUTS prevalence and incidence rates and their increase over time and age-related associations. Each prevalence may be increasing due to an increase in BPH/LUTS disease awareness and diagnosis, the increasing lifespan among men, or a change in treatment-seeking behavior among aging men in order to increase their quality of life.

REFERENCES

1. Roehrborn CG. Benign prostatic hyperplasia: an overview. Rev Urol 2005;7(Suppl 9):S3–s14.
2. Abrams P, Cardozo L, Fall M, et al. The standardisation of terminology in lower urinary tract function: report from the standardisation sub-committee of the International Continence Society. Urology 2003; 61:37–49.
3. Maserejian NN, Chen S, Chiu GR, et al. Incidence of lower urinary tract symptoms in a population-based study of men and women. Urology 2013;82:560–4.
4. Litman HJ, McKinlay JB. The future magnitude of urological symptoms in the USA: projections using the Boston Area Community Health survey. BJU Int 2007;100:820–5.
5. Auffenberg GB, Helfand BT, McVary KT. Established medical therapy for benign prostatic hyperplasia. Urol Clin North Am 2009;36:443–59. v-vi.
6. Anderson JB, Roehrborn CG, Schalken JA, et al. The progression of benign prostatic hyperplasia: examining the evidence and determining the risk. Eur Urol 2001;39:390–9.
7. McNeal J. Pathology of benign prostatic hyperplasia. Insight into etiology. Urol Clin North Am 1990; 17:477–86.
8. Park HJ, Won JE, Sorsaburu S, et al. Urinary tract symptoms (LUTS) secondary to benign prostatic hyperplasia (BPH) and LUTS/BPH with erectile dysfunction in Asian men: a systematic review

focusing on Tadalafil. World J Mens Health 2013;31: 193–207.

9. Rhodes PR, Krogh RH, Bruskewitz RC. Impact of drug therapy on benign prostatic hyperplasia-specific quality of life. Urology 1999; 53:1090–8.

10. Barry MJ, Fowler FJ Jr, O'Leary MP, et al. Measuring disease-specific health status in men with benign prostatic hyperplasia. Measurement Committee of The American Urological Association. Med Care 1995;33:As145–AS155.

11. Barry MJ, Fowler FJ Jr, O'Leary MP, et al. The American Urological Association symptom index for benign prostatic hyperplasia. The Measurement Committee of the American Urological Association. J Urol 1992;148:1549–57 [discussion: 1564].

12. Egan KB, Burnett AL, McVary KT, et al. The co-occurring syndrome-coexisting erectile dysfunction and benign prostatic hyperplasia and their clinical correlates in aging men: results from the national health and nutrition examination survey. Urology 2015;86:570–80.

13. Roehrborn CG, Nuckolls JG, Wei JT, et al. The benign prostatic hyperplasia registry and patient survey: study design, methods and patient baseline characteristics. BJU Int 2007;100:813–9.

14. Kirby M, Chapple C, Jackson G, et al. Erectile dysfunction and lower urinary tract symptoms: a consensus on the importance of co-diagnosis. Int J Clin Pract 2013;67:606–18.

15. Kristal AR, Arnold KB, Schenk JM, et al. Race/ethnicity, obesity, health related behaviors and the risk of symptomatic benign prostatic hyperplasia: results from the prostate cancer prevention trial. J Urol 2007;177:1395–400 [quiz: 1591].

16. Parsons JK. Lifestyle factors, benign prostatic hyperplasia, and lower urinary tract symptoms. Curr Opin Urol 2011;21:1–4.

17. Wei JT, Calhoun E, Jacobsen SJ. Urologic diseases in America project: benign prostatic hyperplasia. J Urol 2005;173:1256–61.

18. Blanker MH, Bohnen AM, Groeneveld FP, et al. Correlates for erectile and ejaculatory dysfunction in older Dutch men: a community-based study. J Am Geriatr Soc 2001;49:436–42.

19. Coyne KS, Kaplan SA, Chapple CR, et al. Risk factors and comorbid conditions associated with lower urinary tract symptoms: EpiLUTS. BJU Int 2009; 103(Suppl 3):24–32.

20. Bosch JL, Hop WC, Kirkels WJ, et al. Natural history of benign prostatic hyperplasia: appropriate case definition and estimation of its prevalence in the community. Urology 1995;46:34–40.

21. Lee AJ, Garraway WM, Simpson RJ, et al. The natural history of untreated lower urinary tract symptoms in middle-aged and elderly men over a period of five years. Eur Urol 1998;34:325–32.

22. Berry SJ, Coffey DS, Walsh PC, et al. The development of human benign prostatic hyperplasia with age. J Urol 1984;132:474–9.

23. Garraway WM, Collins GN, Lee RJ. High prevalence of benign prostatic hypertrophy in the community. Lancet 1991;338:469–71.

24. Meigs JB, Mohr B, Barry MJ, et al. Risk factors for clinical benign prostatic hyperplasia in a community-based population of healthy aging men. J Clin Epidemiol 2001;54:935–44.

25. Sarma AV, Jacobson DJ, McGree ME, et al. A population based study of incidence and treatment of benign prostatic hyperplasia among residents of Olmsted County, Minnesota: 1987 to 1997. J Urol 2005;173:2048–53.

26. Kupelian V, Wei JT, O'Leary MP, et al. Prevalence of lower urinary tract symptoms and effect on quality of life in a racially and ethnically diverse random sample: the Boston Area Community Health (BACH) Survey. Arch Intern Med 2006; 166:2381–7.

27. Da Silva FC. Benign prostatic hyperplasia: natural evolution versus medical treatment. Eur Urol 1997; 32(Suppl 2):34–7.

28. Napalkov P, Maisonneuve P, Boyle P. Worldwide patterns of prevalence and mortality from benign prostatic hyperplasia. Urology 1995;46:41–6.

29. De Marzo AM, Marchi VL, Epstein JI, et al. Proliferative inflammatory atrophy of the prostate: implications for prostatic carcinogenesis. Am J Pathol 1999;155:1985–92.

30. Girman CJ, Jacobsen SJ, Guess HA, et al. Natural history of prostatism: relationship among symptoms, prostate volume and peak urinary flow rate. J Urol 1995;153:1510–5.

31. Chute CG, Panser LA, Girman CJ, et al. The prevalence of prostatism: a population-based survey of urinary symptoms. J Urol 1993;150:85–9.

32. McVary KT. BPH: epidemiology and comorbidities. Am J Manag Care 2006;12:S122–8.

33. Bosch JL, Hop WC, Kirkels WJ, et al. The International Prostate Symptom Score in a community-based sample of men between 55 and 74 years of age: prevalence and correlation of symptoms with age, prostate volume, flow rate and residual urine volume. Br J Urol 1995;75:622–30.

34. Sagnier PP, MacFarlane G, Richard F, et al. Results of an epidemiological survey using a modified American Urological Association symptom index for benign prostatic hyperplasia in France. J Urol 1994;151:1266–70.

35. Chicharro-Molero JA, Burgos-Rodriguez R, Sanchez-Cruz JJ, et al. Prevalence of benign prostatic hyperplasia in Spanish men 40 years old or older. J Urol 1998;159:878–82.

36. Rhodes T, Girman CJ, Jacobsen SJ, et al. Longitudinal prostate growth rates during 5 years in randomly

selected community men 40 to 79 years old. J Urol 1999;161:1174–9.

37. Bushman W. Etiology, epidemiology, and natural history of benign prostatic hyperplasia. Urol Clin North Am 2009;36:403–15, v.

38. Vesely S, Knutson T, Damber JE, et al. Relationship between age, prostate volume, prostate-specific antigen, symptom score and uroflowmetry in men with lower urinary tract symptoms. Scand J Urol Nephrol 2003;37:322–8.

39. Ezz el Din K, Kiemeney LA, de Wildt MJ, et al. Correlation between uroflowmetry, prostate volume, postvoid residue, and lower urinary tract symptoms as measured by the International Prostate Symptom Score. Urology 1996;48:393–7.

40. Van Den Eeden SK, Shan J, Jacobsen SJ, et al. Evaluating racial/ethnic disparities in lower urinary tract symptoms in men. J Urol 2012;187:185–9.

41. Wei JT, Schottenfeld D, Cooper K, et al. The natural history of lower urinary tract symptoms in black American men: relationships with aging, prostate size, flow rate and bothersomeness. J Urol 2001; 165:1521–5.

42. Jin B, Turner L, Zhou Z, et al. Ethnicity and migration as determinants of human prostate size. J Clin Endocrinol Metab 1999;84:3613–9.

43. Masumori N, Tsukamoto T, Kumamoto Y, et al. Japanese men have smaller prostate volumes but comparable urinary flow rates relative to American men: results of community based studies in 2 countries. J Urol 1996;155:1324–7.

44. Platz EA, Smit E, Curhan GC, et al. Prevalence of and racial/ethnic variation in lower urinary tract symptoms and noncancer prostate surgery in U.S. men. Urology 2002;59:877–83.

45. Verhamme KM, Dieleman JP, Bleumink GS, et al. Incidence and prevalence of lower urinary tract symptoms suggestive of benign prostatic hyperplasia in primary care—the Triumph project. Eur Urol 2002;42:323–8.

46. Platz EA, Joshu CE, Mondul AM, et al. Incidence and progression of lower urinary tract symptoms in a large prospective cohort of United States men. J Urol 2012;188:496–501.

47. Clifford GM, Logie J, Farmer RD. How do symptoms indicative of BPH progress in real life practice? The UK experience. Eur Urol 2000;38(Suppl 1):48–53.

48. Logie JW, Clifford GM, Farmer RD, et al. Lower urinary tract symptoms suggestive of benign prostatic obstruction–Triumph: the role of general practice databases. Eur Urol 2001;39(Suppl 3):42–7.

49. Tsukamoto T, Kumamoto Y, Masumori N, et al. Prevalence of prostatism in Japanese men in a community-based study with comparison to a similar American study. J Urol 1995;154:391–5.

50. Guess HA. Benign prostatic hyperplasia: antecedents and natural history. Epidemiol Rev 1992;14: 131–53.

51. Nickel JC. Benign prostatic hyperplasia: does prostate size matter? Rev Urol 2003;5(Suppl 4):S12–7.

52. Platz EA, Kawachi I, Rimm EB, et al. Race, ethnicity and benign prostatic hyperplasia in the health professionals follow-up study. J Urol 2000;163:490–5.

Diagnostic Work-Up of Lower Urinary Tract Symptoms

Sarah L. Hecht, MD, Jason C. Hedges, MD, PhD*

KEYWORDS

- Benign prostatic hyperplasia • Prostatic enlargement • Bladder outlet obstruction • Diagnosis
- Testing • Work-up • Lower urinary tract symptoms

KEY POINTS

- The focus of the initial evaluation of LUTS should be to assess symptomatology and rule out etiologies other than prostatic enlargement.
- Algorithms for the evaluation of LUTS rely largely on expert opinion.
- All patients presenting with LUTS should undergo a medical history, physical examination with DRE, and urinalysis.
- Data regarding the benefits of invasive testing including pressure-flow studies, prostate ultrasound, and endoscopy are lacking and mixed.
- The extent of the diagnostic work-up should depend on symptom severity and planned intervention.

INTRODUCTION

Benign prostatic hyperplasia (BPH) is a histologic diagnosis defined by proliferation of benign prostatic stromal and epithelial tissue. It can lead to benign prostatic enlargement and subsequent bladder outlet obstruction and/or lower urinary tract symptoms (LUTS). Most patients with BPH presenting to their urologist come with a chief complaint of LUTS.[1] The goal of the initial work-up is two-fold: assess the severity of the patient's symptoms and rule out alternative etiologies. Broadly speaking, the extent of the work-up should depend on the extent of symptoms, the suspected cause, and the planned therapy. Fortunately non-BPH causes of LUTS are usually easily identified by history; physical examination; and inexpensive, noninvasive testing. For patients in whom the diagnosis remains unclear after initial work-up, additional diagnostic testing may be helpful.

Given that BPH is a progressive disease, a secondary goal is to identify patients at risk of rapid symptomatic progression and of

complications of BPH, because these patients may decide to pursue more aggressive therapies early on. Complications of BPH include urinary retention, gross hematuria, recurrent urinary tract infection (UTI), bladder stones, and bladder decompensation (diverticula, decreased contractility, hypercontractility, hypertrophy with increased voiding pressures, and obstructive nephropathy). Patients who present with complications of BPH are subject to a different diagnostic algorithm than those presenting with isolated LUTS.

PATIENT HISTORY
Symptom Score

A validated assessment of LUTS is uniformly recommended in the initial work-up of LUTS, both as an objective assessment of symptoms and a quantifiable metric by which to measure efficacy of treatment. The International Prostate Symptom Score (IPSS) is a scoring system originally developed by the American Urologic

Urology, Oregon Health & Science University, 3303 Southwest Bond Avenue, CH10U, Portland, OR 97239, USA
* Corresponding author.
E-mail address: hedgesja@ohsu.edu

Urol Clin N Am 43 (2016) 299–309
http://dx.doi.org/10.1016/j.ucl.2016.04.002
0094-0143/16/$ – see front matter © 2016 Elsevier Inc. All rights reserved.

Association (AUA), and is now the standard assessment in the United States.[2,3] In this questionnaire, seven voiding symptoms are rated on a five-point Likert scale, followed by a quality of life score. Symptom scores are summed and classified as mild (0–7), moderate (8–19), or severe (20–35). Although the IPSS is internally consistent and reliable, there are certainly limitations. First and foremost IPSS does not diagnose BPH and does not determine treatment, which is guided primarily by quality of life score and complications of BPH. The validity of the self-administered IPSS varies across socioeconomic class.[4] Other validated scoring systems do exist (eg, Danish Prostate Symptom Score, BPH Impact Index); however, these are less ubiquitous in North America.[5]

Frequency-Volume Charts

Frequency-volume charts, or voiding diaries, are simple to complete, inexpensive, and can provide useful objective insights into a patient's voiding history. These can serve as an adjunct to the IPSS, and tend to be more accurate that patient recall.[6,7] Although there is no standard diary protocol data suggest that a voiding diary should last at least 3 days, with the goal of being long enough to avoid sampling error but short enough to optimize compliance.[8–10] The AUA guideline on the management of BPH suggests that frequency-volume charts be used in patients with nocturia as the dominant symptom to help identify patients with isolated nocturnal polyuria or excessive fluid intake. Polyuria, defined in the AUA guidelines as urine output greater than 3 L daily, or nocturnal polyuria, defined as more than one-third of urine output during the night, should be approached initially with lifestyle modification.[11]

Additional History

In addition to an assessment of voiding symptoms, the patient interview must include a directed history regarding alternative causes of voiding dysfunction. Specific additional areas to discuss when evaluating a man with LUTS include a history of UTI, hematuria, diabetes, spine and neurologic disease, prior urinary retention, and sleep disorders including sleep apnea. Any prior urologic history including urinary catheterization and instrumentation should be elucidated, as should risk factors for urethral stricture disease including prior trauma or sexually transmitted infections. A smoking history is important to assess the risk for bladder cancer and because nicotine is a bladder irritant.[12] Medications and supplements should be reviewed in detail, with particular attention to

medications that increase outflow resistance (eg, α-sympathomimetic agents) or reduce bladder contractility (eg, anticholinergics).

PHYSICAL EXAMINATION

The physical examination of patients with LUTS suspected to be caused by BPH should include the following:

1. Abdominal examination: to evaluate for a palpably distended bladder
2. Genitourinary examination: evaluate meatal stenosis, phimosis, urethral discharge, lichen sclerosis (which can be associated with stricture disease), and urethral mass
3. Focused neurologic examination: including motor and sensory function of the perineum and lower limbs
4. Digital rectal examination (DRE): to evaluate sphincter tone, prostate nodules, tenderness or bogginess of the prostate, rectal masses, and to give an estimate of prostate size

Digital estimation of prostate size is notoriously inaccurate, although one can generally distinguish prostates less than 50 g from those greater than 50 g.[13] Training with a dedicated model can improve accuracy.[14–16] Moreover, prostate size does not correlate well with symptom severity, degree of urodynamic obstruction, or treatment outcomes.[17,18] Still, given that gland size portends a greater risk of BPH progression and may guide pharmacologic or surgical approach, a general estimate of size based on DRE can be valuable.

IMAGING AND ADDITIONAL TESTING

Some basic, noninvasive testing is recommended in all patients. Urologists may pursue additional imaging and additional testing in the work-up of LUTS when invasive therapies are being considered, or where there is suspicion that the patients' symptoms are not caused by BPH.

Urine Studies

Urinalysis with urine microscopy is recommended for all men presenting with LUTS.[11,19–21] Although serious urinary tract pathology is rarely detected, urinalysis is an innocuous, inexpensive, simple to perform test, and the benefits clearly outweigh the harm. It may reveal the following:

- UTI: Detecting UTI is important in men with LUTS for two reasons. UTI can mimic LUTS, and a symptom assessment should be repeated once the UTI is treated. Moreover, recurrent UTIs in patients with BPH and bladder outlet obstruction is an indication to pursue invasive treatments, even in the setting of minimal LUTS.

- Glucosuria, proteinuria: Occasionally, diabetes is detected by the presence of glucose in the urine. Additionally, protein in the urine may be an early indicator of medical renal disease. Polyuria caused by either diabetes or a renal concentrating defect may mimic LUTS caused by BPH.
- Hematuria: Detection of microhematuria prompts a microhematuria work-up, which may reveal alternative etiologies of LUTS including urothelial cancer or, more rarely, distal ureteral stones. Even without microhematuria, consideration may be given to urine cytology in men with severe irritable symptoms and dysuria, particularly if there is a history of smoking. Bladder cancer and carcinoma in situ notoriously mimics the storage symptoms of BPH, and a missed diagnosis is potentially catastrophic.

Serum Creatinine

Historically, measurement of serum creatinine has been recommended in the initial work-up of BPH to rule out obstructive uropathy.[22,23] Because the incidence of baseline renal insufficiency seems to be no higher in the BPH population than the population at large, the most recent iteration of the AUA guidelines no longer recommends obtaining serum creatinine in patients whose initial work-up reveals LUTS only. Analysis of the MTOPS trial data shows that the risk of developing de novo renal failure in men with LUTS is minimal (<1%).[24] A model of shared decision making is suggested when it comes to initial testing beyond urinalysis, with the thought that progression of BPH will be detected with yearly re-evaluation of symptoms. For patients with LUTS who have a history of hypertension or diabetes, there does seem to be an increased risk for renal disease and

physicians should consider obtaining serum creatinine in these patients.[25] Moreover, given that patients with elevated serum creatinine suffer more perioperative complications, it is reasonable to check creatinine in all patients before surgical intervention.[26]

Prostate-Specific Antigen

Prostate cancer may present with LUTS by producing bladder outlet obstruction similar to benign prostatic enlargement. In men with a life expectancy of at least 10 years, a diagnosis of prostate cancer may well alter the treatment of their voiding symptoms. Moreover, LUTS caused by obstruction from prostate cancer may respond differently to standard treatment approaches. Prostate-specific antigen (PSA) testing should be offered to patients who have at least a 10-year life expectancy, and for whom a diagnosis of prostate cancer would change management.[10,19,21,27] As with all patients being offered PSA testing for prostate cancer screening, a thorough discussion of limitations of the test, alternative causes of PSA elevation, and the risks and benefits of prostate biopsy should be held.

Given that BPH is a source of elevated PSA, there is significant overlap between the serum PSA values of men with BPH and with early prostate cancer; more than one-quarter of patients with histologically proven BPH have a serum PSA value greater than 4.0 ng/mL.[22] PSA velocity, percent free PSA, and, for patients who undergo transrectal ultrasound, PSA density may help improve the specificity of PSA in detecting prostate cancer in men with BPH.

In the absence of malignancy, PSA is a useful surrogate of prostate size. In a study of nearly 4500 men with BPH and without prostate cancer Roehrborn and colleagues[28] demonstrated an age-dependent, log-linear relationship between PSA and prostate volume, with a steeper rise in prostate volume per increase in PSA as men get

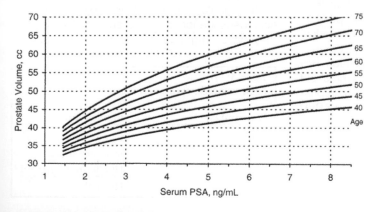

Fig. 1. Predicting prostate volume based on age and PSA. Nomogram developed by Roehrborn and colleagues based on the analysis of PSA and prostate volume in nearly 4500 patients with BPH without prostate cancer. The authors suggest the predicted prostate volume has an error margin of roughly ± 5 mL. (From Roehrborn CG, Boyle P, Gould AL, et al. Serum prostate-specific antigen as a predictor of prostate volume in men with benign prostatic hyperplasia. Urology 1999;53(3):581–9; with permission.)

older (**Fig. 1**). Their data reveal that age-specific thresholds for detecting men with prostate glands exceeding 30 mL (within the realm of responsiveness to 5α-reductase inhibitors) are greater than or equal to 1.3 ng/mL, greater than or equal to 1.5 ng/mL, and greater than or equal to 1.7 ng/mL in men with BPH in their 50s, 60s, and 70s, respectively. This relationship was confirmed by a retrospective analysis of more than 1800 Dutch patients that shows that 89% of men with PSA greater than 1.5 ng/mL have a prostate volume greater than 30 mL, and by the MTOPS data, which show that PSA greater than 1.5 ng/mL represents a prostate volume of greater than or equal to 30 mL regardless of age.[29,30]

Evidence also suggests that PSA can predict the risk of BPH progression, the likelihood of response to 5α-reductase inhibitors, the need for surgical intervention, and the risk of urinary retention.[31–33] Urologists should note that in men with BPH already treated with 5α-reductase inhibitors PSA values can be reduced by 40% to 50% after 6 months of therapy and may be difficult to interpret in the absence of a pretreatment baseline.[34] For this reason, urologists must obtain a baseline PSA before initiating therapy with 5α-reductase inhibitors.

Postvoid Residual Urine Volume

Postvoid residual (PVR) urine volumes are typically assessed by noninvasive transabdominal ultrasound. This is another rapid, noninvasive, inexpensive test with few downsides, although retest measurement variability yields repeated measurements prudent. Note that alternative sources of pelvic fluid, such as ascites or a reservoir for an inflatable penile prosthesis, fool the machine. In patients with bladder outlet obstruction caused by BPH, residual urine is useful to assess and follow the degree of using. PVR cannot distinguish between obstructive urinary retention and myogenic or neurogenic urinary retention, but can to some extent distinguish obstruction from isolated overactive bladder, because patients with isolated overactive bladder should have low residual urines.

A precise definition for urinary retention has been notoriously elusive, and as such a threshold PVR has never been agreed on. There is a surprising lack of clear correlation between elevated PVR and episodes of acute urinary retention (AUR) or the need for invasive treatment. In their study of nearly 1000 patients with BPH treated with watchful waiting or α-blockers, Mochtar and colleagues[35] found PVR to be unhelpful in predicting the risk of AUR, and only patients with PVRs

greater than 300 mL were at increased risk of requiring invasive therapy. Conversely, Klarskov and colleagues[36] found that of men with AUR, a PVR greater than 500 mL increased the risk of recurrent AUR by a factor of 3.6. In men with lesser residual volumes, it has been difficult to show a relation between PVR and any urinary outcome.[37] As noted by Kaplan and colleagues,[38] the lack of correlation with PVR may merely represent the exclusion of men in many studies with PVR greater than 150 mL. There are little data to suggest that elevated PVR should prompt upper tract imaging to evaluate hydronephrosis, because hydronephrosis is thought to result more from ureteral obstruction from BPH and/or from a low-compliance bladder.[39]

Peak Urine Flow Rate

Like residual volume, flow rate is a measure of bladder and outlet function, and cannot definitively distinguish between the two. It is generally accepted that a maximum flow rate less than 10 mL/s indicates a high probability of obstruction, whereas a flow rate greater than 15 mL/s indicates a low probability.[40,41] **Table 1** outlines general maximum flow rate values and their implications; however, flow rates must be interpreted in the setting of voided volume and age. For men with suspected bladder outlet obstruction, the International Continence Society has published a nomogram that groups men into three categories (obstructed, unobstructed, and equivocal) based on maximum flow rate and maximum detrusor pressure, although this requires pressure-flow studies for evaluation (**Fig. 2**).[42] The Olmsted Community study used a cutoff of 12 mL/s, and showed that men with peak urine flow rates below this had nearly three times the risk of surgery and AUR than those with higher flow rates.[43] Conversely, in the MTOPS study a peak flow rate less than 10.6 mL per second was not predictive of AUR in placebo-treated subjects (**Fig. 3**).[44]

Although flow rates are limited by diurnal variation, dependence on age, and volume voided, they have long been used as a surrogate for

Table 1		
Peak urine flow rates in men		
Q_{max} (mL/s)		**Implication**
<10		Likely obstructed
10–15		Indeterminate
>15		Likely unobstructed
20–25		Normal

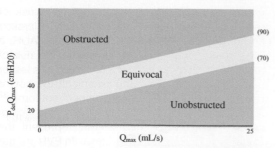

Fig. 2. International Continence Society provisional nomogram. Patients are divided into three classes (unobstructed, equivocal, and obstructed) based on the bladder outlet obstruction index (BOOI), a function of detrusor pressure at maximum flow rate ($P_{det}Q_{max}$) and maximum flow rate (Q_{max}). (*Adapted from* Abrams P. Bladder outlet obstruction index, bladder contractility index and bladder voiding efficiency: three simple indices to define bladder voiding function. BJU Int 1999;84:14; with permission.)

obstruction. Many BPH trials used flow rates cut-offs of 10 to 15 mL/s as entry criteria. Because of intraindividual variability and the volume dependency of flow rate, the European Association of Urology and AUA guidelines suggest obtaining two flow rates with a void volume greater than 150 mL.[11,19] Results can be used to predict the need for invasive therapy, and as an additional

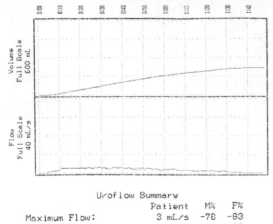

Uroflow Summary

	Patient	M%	F%
Maximum Flow:	3 mL/s	-78	-83
Average Flow:	2 mL/s	-78	-83
Voiding Time:	84 s	-286	-338
Flow Time:	84 s		
Time To Maximum Flow:	23 s	-121	-180
Voided Volume:	208 mL		

Fig. 3. Uroflowmetry. Urine flow study showing a prolonged voiding time, flattened curve, and low maximum flow rate (3 mL/s) consistent with bladder outlet obstruction. This is an adequate study with a voided volume greater than 150 mL. A similar curve may be seen with poor detrusor function.

objective metric of disease progression or response to therapy.

Pressure-Flow Studies

Pressure-flow studies represent the gold standard in diagnosis of bladder outlet obstruction. The distinction between poor detrusor contractility and outlet obstruction is made by measuring detrusor pressures and flow rate during maximum flow. High pressure with low flow defines urodynamic obstruction (**Fig. 4**). In 1994, Abrams[45] argued that pressure-flow studies should be conducted in all patients with suspected LUTS caused by BPH on the following basis: cost-savings of averted ineffective therapies, low complication rates, and no alternative testing can definitively establish a diagnosis. Nevertheless, pressure-flow studies are invasive, expensive, and updated guidelines generally do not recommend these in the work-up of BPH. Abrams himself has moved to recommend pressure-flow studies only for men with peak urine flow rates greater than 10 mL/s to clarify the diagnosis.[21] The benefit of this invasive work-up is that a definitive diagnosis of obstruction should reliably predict response to surgical therapy.

Indeed, there are data to support this logic. Rodrigues and colleagues[46] evaluated 253 patients who elected to undergo transurethral prostate resection as treatment of their LUTS. All patients underwent preoperative and postoperative urodynamic evaluation and IPSS assessment. Nearly half of patients were not urodynamically obstructed and could not be distinguished from obstructed patients based on IPSS or quality of life score. The entire obstructed group demonstrated marked improvement on postoperative urodynamics and IPSS, whereas the nonobstructed group did not. Moreover, clinical benefit increased with the severity of obstruction. The authors concluded that urodynamic obstruction precisely predicted good responses to surgical therapy in obstructed patients and poor outcomes in nonobstructed patients. Alternative therapies (antichlolinergics, bladder training, biofeedback) are recommended for patients with severe LUTS without demonstrated obstruction on pressure-flow studies.[21]

Other investigators have not found pressure-flow studies so useful. To create a model predicting outcomes following prostate resection, Kanik and colleagues[47] found that urodynamic variables added no predictive value on top of age and peak flow rate. Moreover, Van Venrooij and colleagues[48] found that urodynamically unobstructed or equivocal men with severe LUTS who underwent prostate resection enjoyed 70% of the symptomatic

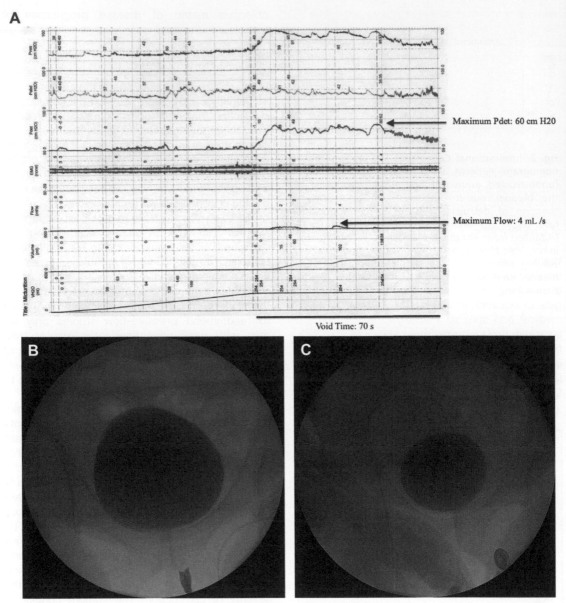

Maximum Pdet: 60 cm H20

Maximum Flow: 4 mL /s

Void Time: 70 s

Fig. 4. Pressure-flow studies. (*A*) The pressure-flow curve demonstrates an obstructed pattern with a coordinated detrusor contraction, elevated voiding pressure (>50 cm H_2O), and low flow rate (<4 mL/s). (*B*) Fluoroscopic image showing a closed bladder neck and prostatic urethra during voiding. (*C*) A patient without bladder outlet obstruction has an open bladder neck and "funnel-shaped" open prostatic urethra during voiding.

improvements of their urodynanmically obstructed counterparts. Han and colleagues[49] similarly found that urodynamically unobstructed men with weak bladder contractility on urodynamics had significant improvement in IPSS, quality of life score, and PVR following transurethral resection of the prostate. This is presumably because of decreased urethral resistance in the setting of poor detrusor function. Taken together, these data suggest that the absence of urodynamic obstruction does not make surgical intervention entirely futile, which

calls into question the clinical utility of performing pressure-flow studies before surgery.

Prostate Ultrasonography

Prostate ultrasound provides the gold standard assessment of size and shape of the prostate. Although not recommended for work-up of isolated LUTS, knowledge of prostate size may predict response to 5α-reductase inhibitors, and knowledge of prostate size and configuration may help guide surgical technique. Classically, prostate size was the deciding factor between transurethral prostate resection and open prostatectomy because of the risk of transurethral resection (TUR) syndrome with prolonged transurethral surgery. Although bipolar transurethral resection of the prostate has largely diminished this risk, prostate size and configuration may still be relevant to the operating surgeon. For instance, a laser procedure may be less desirable in a patient with a large median lobe because of risk of injuring the ureteral orifices. Urolift, a new minimally invasive surgical therapy, has only been studied in men with prostates less than 80 mL. Its efficacy in larger glands is unproved, and it cannot be used in the presence of a median lobe.[50]

Transabdominal ultrasound has been gaining traction as a noninvasive alternative to transrectal ultrasound. In particular, intravesical prostatic protrusion has been identified as a promising surrogate of obstruction and predictor of response to medical and surgical therapies.[51–53] Intravesical prostatic protrusion is measured in millimeters from the bladder neck in a midsagittal view and is graded by severity as grade I (<5 mm), grade II (5–10 mm), and grade III (>10 mm) **(Fig. 5)**.[54] Certainly these data are preliminary, but if proven

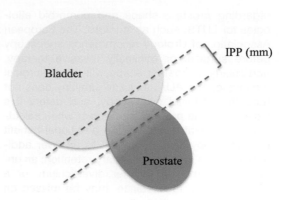

Fig. 5. Intravesical prostatic protrusion (IPP). A schematic showing the measurement of IPP, graded by severity as grade I (<5 mm), grade II (5–10 mm), and grade III (>10 mm).

durable transabdominal ultrasound may provide urologists with an additional inexpensive, noninvasive tool in the work-up of LUTS.

Endoscopy

As with prostate ultrasound, cystourethroscopy is generally not recommended in the initial evaluation of LUTS but can provide valuable information

Table 2
American Urologic Association Guidelines

	Recommended	Optional	Not Recommended
History	X	—	—
Symptom score	X	—	—
Voiding diary	—	X[a]	—
Physical, including DRE	X	—	—
Urinalysis	X	—	—
Serum creatinine	—	—	X
PSA	—	X[b]	—
PVR	—	X	—
Flow rate	—	X[c]	—
Pressure-flow studies	—	—	X[d]
Prostate ultrasound	—	X	—
Cystoscopy	—	—	X[e]
Upper tract imaging	—	—	X[f]

[a] When nocturia is present.
[b] If life expectancy is >10 years and if diagnosis of prostate cancer would modify management approach.
[c] Obtain two flow rates with >150 mL voided volume.
[d] Consider in patients with Q_{max} >10 mL/s to establish diagnosis of obstruction, given higher failure rates of surgery in the absence of obstruction.
[e] Recommended if considering treatment alternatives, such as transurethral incision or microwave therapy.
[f] Recommended only if patients have a history of hematuria, upper tract infection, urolithiasis, renal insufficiency, recent-onset nocturnal enuresis.

Data from McVary KT, Roehrborn CG, Avins AL, et al. Update on AUA Guideline on the management of benign prostatic hyperplasia. J Urol 2011;185(5):1793–803.

regarding prostate shape and comorbid etiologies for LUTS, such as stricture. The European Association of Urology recommends endoscopy before surgical or minimally invasive therapy, particularly if prostate shape will affect surgical technique. The AUA guideline similarly does not recommend initial cystoscopy, and defers this work-up to the practicing urologist when selecting a treatment approach. An additional benefit of cystoscopy is the potential to uncover additional causes of LUTS or urinary retention; an unexpected tumor, a bladder diverticulum, or a bladder stone, for instance, may be missed on standard initial work-up. Anecdotally, the appearance of the bladder may give clues as to the cause of LUTS (ie, a heavily trabeculated bladder may indicate long-standing obstruction), although there is essentially no data to correlate such cystoscopic findings with postoperative outcomes.

Additional Imaging

In the absence of other indications, imaging studies, such as renal ultrasonography, intravenous urography, computed tomography, and MRI, are not recommended in the work-up of LUTS because of their low yield, high up-front costs, and the downstream costs of incidental findings.[55] Upper tract imaging should be considered in patients with elevated creatinine, markedly elevated PVR urine, upper tract infection, history of stones, and hematuria, and in patients with neurologic disease and concern for high-pressure voiding. Renal ultrasound is the initial modality of choice given that it is inexpensive, noninvasive, and lacks radiation.

GUIDELINE OVERVIEW

Tables 2–4 show a tabular overview of the guidelines from the American, European, and Canadian urologic associations and their recommendations

---

Table 3
European Association of Urology

	Recommended	Optional	Not Recommended
History	X[a]	—	—
Symptom score	X	—	—
Voiding diary	X[b]	—	—
Physical, including DRE	X	—	—
Urinalysis	X[a]	—	—
Serum creatinine	—	X[c]	—
PSA	—	X[d]	—
PVR	X	—	—
Flow rate	—	X[e]	—
Pressure-flow studies	—	X[f]	—
Prostate ultrasound	—	X[g]	—
Cystoscopy	—	X[h]	—
Upper tract imaging	—	X[i]	—

[a] Mandatory.
[b] Recommended prominent storage component or nocturia.
[c] Mandatory if renal impairment is suspected clinically, hydronephrosis, or before surgery.
[d] Recommended only if diagnosis of prostate cancer will change management or if PSA can assist in decision making for patients at risk of benign prostatic enlargement progression.
[e] Recommended before initiating treatment.
[f] Recommended for all men who have failed prior invasive treatment of LUTS and before surgery in the following situations: (1) if the voided volume is <150 mL or Q_{max} >15 mL/s before surgical intervention particularly in the elderly to document the presence of benign prostatic obstruction (BPO), (2) younger men (eg, <50 years), (3) elderly men (>80 years), (4) PVR >300 mL, (5) suspicion of neurogenic bladder dysfunction; (6) after radical pelvic surgery; (7) previous unsuccessful invasive treatment.
[g] Recommended before surgical therapy and before medical therapy if it assists choice of the appropriate drug.
[h] Recommended in patients with suspected bladder or urethral pathology, and/or before surgery if findings may change treatment.
[i] Recommended for men with large PVR, hematuria, history of urolithiasis.
 Data from Gratzke C, Bachmann A, Descazeaud A, et al. EAU Guidelines on the assessment of non-neurogenic male lower urinary tract symptoms including benign prostatic obstruction. Eur Urol 2015;67(6):1099–109.

Table 4
Canadian Urological Association

	Recommended	Optional	Not Recommended
History	X[a]	—	—
Symptom score	X	—	—
Voiding diary	—	X	—
Physical, including DRE	X[a]	—	—
Urinalysis	X[a]	—	—
Serum creatinine	—	X	—
PSA	X	—	—
PVR	—	X	—
Flow rate	—	X	—
Pressure-flow studies	—	—	X
Prostate ultrasound	—	—	X
Cystoscopy	—	—	X
Upper tract imaging	—	—	X
Urine cytology	—	—	X[b]

[a] Mandatory.
[b] Optional if irritative symptoms are a significant component of LUTS.
Data from Nickel JC, Méndez-Probst CE, Whelan TF, et al. 2010 Update: guidelines for the management of benign prostatic hyperplasia. Can Urol Assoc J 2010;4(5):310–6.

for the initial work-up of LUTS. Some tests not recommended in the initial work-up do have conditional indications, which are delineated.

SUMMARY

The recommended work-up of LUTS has evolved. The goal of the work-up is to establish the severity and cause of LUTS and to predict with certainty which patients will respond to which treatments. Multiple clinical guidelines exist to help guide urologists in their decision-making. All patients need a medical history with a validated symptom score, a physical examination with a DRE, and a urinalysis. PSA, PVR, and peak urine flow rate provide additional information at little cost. For more invasive testing high-level data are lacking, and guidelines defer to the practicing urologist. The holy grail of the LUTS work-up, a perfect predictor of who will and who will not respond to specific therapies, remains elusive. With current tools, even the most extensive work-up is imperfect, and thus the attempt to balance the costs versus the benefits of invasive testing.

REFERENCES

1. Hutchison A, Farmer R, Chapple C, et al. Characteristics of patients presenting with LUTS/BPH in six European countries. Eur Urol 2006;50(3):555–62.

2. McNicholas TA, Kirby RS, Lepor H. Evaluation and nonsurgical management of benign prostatic hyperplasia. In: Wein AJ, Kavoussi LR, Novick AC, et al, editors. Campbell-Walsh urology. 10th edition. Philadelphia: Elsevier Saunders; 2011. p. 2611–54.

3. Barry MJ, Fowler FJ, O'Leary MP, et al. The American Urological Association symptom index for benign prostatic hyperplasia. The Measurement Committee of the American Urological Association. J Urol 1992;148(5):1549–57.

4. Johnson TV, Schoenberg ED, Abbasi A, et al. Assessment of the performance of the American Urological Association Symptom Score in 2 distinct patient populations. J Urol 2009;181(1):230–7.

5. Kingery L, Martin ML, Naegeli AN, et al. Content validity of the benign prostatic hyperplasia impact index (BII); a measure of how urinary trouble and problems associated with BPH may impact the patient. Int J Clin Pract 2012;66(9):883–90.

6. van Haarst EP, Bosch JL, Heldeweg EA. The International Prostate Symptom Score overestimates nocturia assessed by frequency-volume charts. J Urol 2012;188(1):211–5.

7. Blanker MH, Bohnen AM, Groeneveld FP, et al. Normal voiding patterns and determinants of increased diurnal and nocturnal voiding frequency in elderly men. J Urol 2000;164(4):1201–5.

8. Yap TL, Cromwell DC, Emberton M. A systematic review of the reliability of frequency-volume charts in urological research and its implications for the optimum chart duration. BJU Int 2007;99(1):9–16.

9. Schick E, Jolivet Tremblay M, Dupont C, et al. Frequency-volume chart: the minimum number of days required to obtain reliable results. Neurourol Urodyn 2003;22(2):92–6.

10. Madersbacher S, Alivizatos G, Nordling J, et al. EAU 2004 guidelines on assessment, therapy and follow-up of men with lower urinary tract symptoms suggestive of benign prostatic obstruction (BPH guidelines). Eur Urol 2004;46(5):547–54.

11. McVary KT, Roehrborn CG, Avins AL, et al. Update on AUA guideline on the management of benign prostatic hyperplasia. J Urol 2011;185(5):1793–803.

12. Kanai A, Andersson K-E. Bladder afferent signaling: recent findings. J Urol 2010;183(4):1288–95.

13. Bosch JL, Bohnen AM, Groeneveld FP. Validity of digital rectal examination and serum prostate specific antigen in the estimation of prostate volume in community-based men aged 50 to 78 years: the Krimpen study. Eur Urol 2004;46(6):753–9.

14. Roehrborn CG, Girman CJ, Rhodes T, et al. Correlation between prostate size estimated by digital rectal examination and measured by transrectal ultrasound. Urology 1997;49(4):548–57.

15. Yanoshak SJ, Roehrborn CG, Girman CJ, et al. Use of a prostate model to assist in training for digital rectal examination. Urology 2000;55(5):690–3.

16. Roehrborn CG, Sech S, Montoya J, et al. Interexaminer reliability and validity of a three-dimensional model to assess prostate volume by digital rectal examination. Urology 2001;57(6):1087–92.

17. Roehrborn CG, Chinn HK, Fulgham PF, et al. The role of transabdominal ultrasound in the preoperative evaluation of patients with benign prostatic hypertrophy. J Urol 1986;135(6):1190–3.

18. Simonsen O, Møller-Madsen B, Dørflinger T, et al. The significance of age on symptoms and urodynamic- and cystoscopic findings in benign prostatic hypertrophy. Urol Res 1987;15(6):355–8.

19. Gratzke C, Bachmann A, Descazeaud A, et al. EAU guidelines on the assessment of non-neurogenic male lower urinary tract symptoms including benign prostatic obstruction. Eur Urol 2015;67(6):1099–109.

20. Nickel JC, Méndez-Probst CE, Whelan TF, et al. 2010 Update: guidelines for the management of benign prostatic hyperplasia. Can Urol Assoc J 2010;4(5):310–6.

21. Abrams P, Chapple C, Khoury S, et al. Evaluation and treatment of lower urinary tract symptoms in older men. J Urol 2009;181(4):1779–87.

22. McConnell JD, Barry MJ, Bruskewitz RC. Benign prostatic hyperplasia: diagnosis and treatment. Agency for Health Care Policy and Research. Clin Pract Guidel Quick Ref Guide Clin 1994;8:1–17.

23. Denis L, McConnell J, Yoshida O, et al. Recommendations of the International Scientific Committee: the evaluation and treatment of lower urinary tract symptoms (LUTS) suggestive of benign prostatic obstruction. In: Denis L, Griffiths K, Khoury S, et al, editors. Proceedings of the 4th international consultation on benign prostatic hyperplasia (BPH). Plymouth (UK): Health Publications; 1998. p. 669–84.

24. McConnell JD, Roehrborn CG, Bautista OM, et al. The long-term effect of doxazosin, finasteride, and combination therapy on the clinical progression of benign prostatic hyperplasia. N Engl J Med 2003; 349(25):2387–98.

25. Hong SK, Lee ST, Jeong SJ, et al. Chronic kidney disease among men with lower urinary tract symptoms due to benign prostatic hyperplasia. BJU Int 2010;105(10):1424–8.

26. Mebust WK, Holtgrewe HL, Cockett AT, et al. Transurethral prostatectomy: immediate and postoperative complications. A cooperative study of 13 participating institutions evaluating 3,885 patients. J Urol 1989;141(2):243–7.

27. Kaplan SA. Update on the American Urological Association guidelines for the treatment of benign prostatic hyperplasia. Rev Urol 2006;8(Suppl 4): S10–7.

28. Roehrborn CG, Boyle P, Gould AL, et al. Serum prostate-specific antigen as a predictor of prostate volume in men with benign prostatic hyperplasia. Urology 1999;53(3):581–9.

29. Mochtar CA, Kiemeney LA, van Riemsdijk MM, et al. Prostate-specific antigen as an estimator of prostate volume in the management of patients with symptomatic benign prostatic hyperplasia. Eur Urol 2003;44(6):695–700.

30. Roehrborn CG, Boyle P, Nickel JC. PSA is a significant predictor of objective parameters in men at risk for BPH progression. J Urol 2003; 169:A1362.

31. Roehrborn CG, Boyle P, Bergner D, et al. Serum prostate-specific antigen and prostate volume predict long-term changes in symptoms and flow rate: results of a four-year, randomized trial comparing finasteride versus placebo. Urology 1999;54(4):662–9.

32. Levitt JM, Slawin KM. Prostate-specific antigen and prostate-specific antigen derivatives as predictors of benign prostatic hyperplasia progression. Curr Prostate Rep 2007;5(1):21–6.

33. Anderson JB, Roehrborn CG, Schalken JA, et al. The progression of benign prostatic hyperplasia: examining the evidence and determining the risk. Eur Urol 2001;39(4):390–9.

34. Marks LS, Andriole GL, Fitzpatrick JM, et al. The interpretation of serum prostate specific antigen in en receiving 5α-reductase inhibitors: a review and clinical recommendations. J Urol 2006;176(3): 868–74.

35. Mochtar CA, Kiemeney LA, van Riemsdijk MM, et al. Post-void residual urine volume is not a good predictor of the need for invasive therapy among patients

with benign prostatic hyperplasia. J Urol 2006;
175(1):213–6.

36. Klarskov P, Andersen JT, Asmussen CF, et al. Symptoms and signs predictive of the voiding pattern after acute urinary retention in men. Scand J Urol Nephrol 2010;21(1):23–8.

37. Roehrborn CG, Kaplan SA. Roehrborn: baseline post-void residual urine volume as a predictor of urinary outcomes in men with BPH in the MTOPS study. J Urol 2005;173(Suppl):443. A1638.

38. Kaplan SA, Wein AJ, Staskin DR, et al. Urinary retention and post-void residual urine in men: separating truth from tradition. J Urol 2008;180(1):47–54.

39. Wu S, Yang Y, Duan J. Urodynamic studies on mechanism of hydronephrosis due to BPH. Chin J Urol 2001;5:20.

40. Reynard JM, Yang Q, Donovan JL, et al. The ICS-"BPH" Study: uroflowmetry, lower urinary tract symptoms and bladder outlet obstruction. BJU Int 1998;82(5):619–23.

41. Scofield S, Kaplan SA. Voiding dysfunction in men: pathophysiology and risk factors. Int J Impot Res 2008;20:S2–10.

42. Abrams P. Bladder outlet obstruction index, bladder contractility index and bladder voiding efficiency: three simple indices to define bladder voiding function. BJU Int 1999;84:14–5.

43. Jacobsen SJ, Jacobson DJ, Girman CJ, et al. Treatment for benign prostatic hyperplasia among community dwelling men: The Olmsted County study of urinary symptoms and health status. J Urol 1999; 162(4):1301–6.

44. Crawford ED, Wilson SS, McConnell JD, et al. Baseline factors as predictors of clinical progression of benign prostatic hyperplasia in men treated with placebo. J Urol 2006;175(4):1422–7.

45. Abrams P. In support of pressure-flow studies for evaluating men with lower urinary tract symptoms. Urology 1994;44(2):153–5.

46. Rodrigues P, Lucon AM, Freire GC, et al. Urodynamic pressure flow studies can predict the clinical outcome after transurethal prostatic resection. J Urol 2001;165(2):499–502.

47. Kanik EA, Erdem E, Abidinoglu D, et al. Can the outcome of transurethral resection of the prostate be predicted preoperatively? Urology 2004;64(2): 302–5.

48. van Venrooij GE, van Melick HH, Boon TA. Comparison of outcomes of transurethral prostate resection in urodynamically obstructed versus selected urodynamically unobstructed or equivocal men. Urology 2003;62(4):672–6.

49. Han DH, Jeong YS, Choo MS, et al. The efficacy of transurethral resection of the prostate in the patients with weak bladder contractility index. Urology 2008; 71(4):657–61.

50. Cantwell AL, Bogache WK, Richardson SF, et al. Multicentre prospective crossover study of the "prostatic urethral lift" for the treatment of lower urinary tract symptoms secondary to benign prostatic hyperplasia. BJU Int 2014;113(4):615–22.

51. Franco G, De Nunzio C, Leonardo C, et al. Ultrasound assessment of intravesical prostatic protrusion and detrusor wall thickness—new standards for noninvasive bladder outlet obstruction diagnosis? J Urol 2010;183(6):2270–4.

52. Cumpanas AA, Botoca M, Minciu R, et al. Intravesical prostatic protrusion can be a predicting factor for the treatment outcome in patients with lower urinary tract symptoms due to benign prostatic obstruction treated with tamsulosin. Urology 2013; 81(4):859–63.

53. Arnolds M, Oelke M. Positioning invasive versus noninvasive urodynamics in the assessment of bladder outlet obstruction. Curr Opin Urol 2009; 19(1):55–62.

54. Chia SJ, Heng CT, Chan SP, et al. Correlation of intravesical prostatic protrusion with bladder outlet obstruction. BJU Int 2003;91(4):371–4.

55. Grossfeld GD, Coakley FV. Benign prostatic hyperplasia: clinical overview and value of diagnostic imaging. Radiol Clin North Am 2000;38(1):31–47.

Alpha-blockers for the Treatment of Benign Prostatic Hyperplasia

Herbert Lepor, MD

KEYWORDS

- Alpha-blockers • BPH • Lower urinary tract symptoms • Medical management BPH

KEY POINTS

- Over the last 2 decades the evolution of alpha-blockers for lower urinary tract symptoms (LUTS)/ benign prostatic hyperplasia (BPH) has been to preserve effectiveness, improve tolerability, and eliminate dose titration.
- Today, alpha-blockers represent the first-line treatment of most men with BPH whereby the primary objective is relief from bothersome LUTS.
- The thought that alpha blockers only improve LUTS by relieving BOO is likely an oversimplification.

The first selective alpha-blocker was approved for the treatment of lower urinary tract symptoms (LUTS)/benign prostatic hyperplasia (BPH) in 1992. The evolution of alpha-blockers for LUTS/ BPH has been to preserve effectiveness and improve tolerability following administration of a single daily dose without requirement for dose titration. Today, alpha-blockers represent the first-line treatment of most men with BPH whereby the primary objective is relief from bothersome LUTS. The proposed mechanism of action, which is to decrease bladder outlet obstruction (BOO) via smooth muscle relaxation, is an oversimplification.

HISTORICAL PERSPECTIVE

The evolution of alpha-blockers for the treatment of BPH represents one of the first triumphs of translational medicine.

In 1975, Caine and colleagues[1] investigated the in vitro smooth muscle contractile properties of tissue strips derived from human prostates. Human prostate tissue was shown to elicit a strong contractile response in the presence of phenylephrine, a potent alpha agonist. At the time, the adrenergic receptors were subclassified simply as alpha and beta. The phenylephrine-induced contraction was inhibited by phenoxybenzamine, a selective inhibitor of alpha adrenoceptors. Based on these experiments, Caine and associates[1] proposed that the pathophysiology of BPH was mediated in part by prostate smooth muscle tension and speculated that the disease would be effectively treated by alpha-blockade.

In 1975 Caine and colleagues[2] published the first study suggesting alpha-blockers were effective for the treatment of BPH. A subsequent randomized placebo-controlled study confirmed that phenoxybenzamine improved both uroflow rates and prostatism, which at the time was the terminology describing LUTS arising from the enlarged prostate.[3] The primary limitation of phenoxybenzamine was the adverse events, including high rates of tiredness, dizziness, impaired ejaculation, nasal stuffiness, and hypotension. The use of phenoxybenzamine never gained widespread use for treating BPH.

NYU Langone Medical Center, NYU School of Medicine, 150 East 32nd Street, 2nd Floor, New York, NY 10016, USA
E-mail address: Herbert.Lepor@nyumc.org

Urol Clin N Am 43 (2016) 311–323
http://dx.doi.org/10.1016/j.ucl.2016.04.009
0094-0143/16/$ – see front matter

DEVELOPMENT OF SELECTIVE ALPHA1 BLOCKERS FOR BENIGN PROSTATIC HYPERPLASIA

In the early 1980s, the alpha adrenoceptors were subclassified into alpha 1 and alpha 2. Lepor and Shapiro[4] were first to characterize both the alpha 1 and alpha 2[5] adrenoceptors in human prostate tissue using radio-ligand binding studies and subsequently observed that the contractile properties of prostate smooth muscle was mediated primarily by the alpha 1 subtype.[6]

Prazosin was one of the first alpha 1 blockers developed for the treatment of hypertension. The first multicenter randomized placebo-controlled trial of any selective alpha 1 blocker for symptomatic BPH was reported my Kirby and colleagues.[7] Prazosin significantly improved both the severity of prostatism and peak flow rate (PFR) compared with placebo.

The primary advantage of prazosin over phenoxybenzamine was better tolerance presumably by eliminating the adverse events mediated by alpha 2 adrenoceptor blockade. Although a legitimate comparative trial between prazosin and phenoxybenzamine was never performed, the effectiveness of the two drugs seems to be comparable. Like phenoxybenzamine, the limitation of prazosin was the first dose effect, which required a dose titration to an effective multiple daily dose. No effort was made to seek Food and Drug Administration (FDA) approval for prazosin for the indication of symptomatic BPH presumably because of the limited patent life and the lack of general interest in developing and bringing to market medical therapy for BPH.

The next major advance in the development of alpha-blockers for the treatment of symptomatic BPH was the availability of long-acting selective alpha 1 blockers, such as terazosin and doxazosin. Both drugs were approved by the FDA for the treatment of hypertension in the 1980s. The longer half-life of both drugs allowed for once-daily dosing.

Terazosin was the first of the long-acting selective alpha 1 blockers to be approved by the FDA for the treatment of symptomatic BPH in 1992. Three randomized multicenter placebo-controlled studies leading to the approval of terazosin showed significant treatment-related decreases in symptom severity and increases in PFR over placebo[8–10] (Fig. 1). The author served as the national principal investigator for the first randomized study comparing placebo, 2, 5, and 10 mg of terazosin.[8] Because of the potential safety concerns associated with administering an antihypertensive drug to normotensive men, all subjects were admitted to a monitored hospital facility for 72 hours. The requirement for 3-day hospital observation greatly limited patient accrual. Eventually, the FDA relaxed the in-hospital monitoring requirement to 24 hours and the study was completed. The titration to fixed-dose study was not powered to show whether differences between the doses were statistically significant, although there was a suggestion that improvement in LUTS was dose dependent. Overall, terazosin was well tolerated. Asthenia/fatigue, postural hypotension, dizziness, and somnolence were the treatment-related adverse events (Table 1).

The FDA required a long-term extension study in order to demonstrate the durability of efficacy.

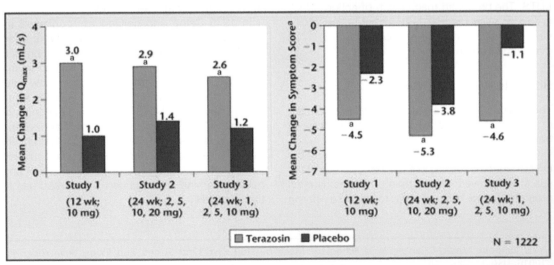

Fig. 1. The effect of terazosin on LUTS and PFR relative to placebo. Q_{max}, maximum urinary flow. [a] $P \leq .05$ versus placebo. (*From* Lepor H. The evolution of alpha-blockers for the treatment of benign prostatic hyperplasia. Rev Urol 2006:8(Suppl 4):53–9; with permission.)

Table 1
Terazosin adverse effects

Adverse Effect	Terazosin (%) (n = 636)	Placebo (%) (n = 360)
Asthenia/fatigue	7.4[a]	3.3
Postural	3.9[a]	0.8
Hypotension		
Dizziness	9.1[a]	4.2
Somnolence	3.6[a]	1.9
Nasal congestion/ rhinitis	1.9[a]	0
Impotence	1.6[a]	0.6

[a] $P \leq .05$ versus placebo.

From Lepor H. The evolution of alpha-blockers for the treatment of benign prostatic hyperplasia. Rev Urol 2006:8(Suppl 4):S3–9; with permission.

Subjects enrolled in the pivotal randomized placebo-controlled studies were given the opportunity to participate in a long-term open-label study that demonstrated durability of efficacy and emergence of no safety issues.[11]

The chemical structure of terazosin and doxazosin are quite similar. It is not surprising that multicenter randomized placebo-controlled FDA registration studies for doxazosin and terazosin were virtually identical as far as treatment-related efficacy and side effects.[12,13] The study designs included a titration to a fixed dose with the dose progressively increasing from 2 mg to 4 mg to 8 mg. The efficacy of these trials comparing placebo, 4 mg, and 8 mg of doxazosin is shown in

Fig. 2. In the titration to fixed dose study, a dose response to doxazosin was not observed. The side effects attributable to doxazosin were fatigue and dizziness (**Table 2**). The FDA approved doxazosin for the treatment of BPH in the mid 1990s.

A long-term open-label study of doxazosin showed durability of efficacy and no emerging new safety issues.[14]

In clinical practice, it is reasonable to assume that nonresponders will choose not to stay on the drug. Therefore, the performance of a drug in randomized placebo-controlled trials underestimates the effectiveness of the drug in clinical practice. MacDiarmid and colleagues[15] provide the most compelling evidence for the dose response to alpha-blockers in clinical practice. Responders to 4 mg daily doxazosin were randomized to remain on 4 mg or to increase the dose to 8 mg. Very significant improvements in both symptom scores and PFR were observed between the 4- and 8-mg doses. This study supported the author's recommendation to titrate both terazosin and doxazosin to the maximal tolerable dose. One of the more troublesome side effects leading to withdrawal of both terazosin and doxazosin was asthenia and dizziness. In order to improve tolerability, a second recommendation was to administer the doses at bedtime.

Tamsulosin was the next alpha 1 blocker to be FDA approved in the United States. Both pivotal registration trials compared daily placebo versus 4 mg and 8 mg tamsulosin.[16,17] The initial dose for all men randomized to tamsulosin was 4 mg with a subsequent titration to the 8-mg dose. Both doses of tamsulosin were superior to

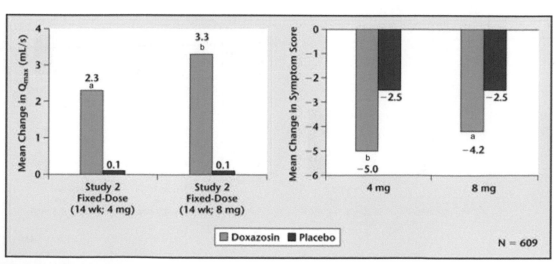

Fig. 2. The effect of doxazosin on LUTS and PFR relative to placebo. [a] $P<.05$ versus placebo; [b] $P = .01$ versus placebo. (*From* Lepor H. The evolution of alpha-blockers for the treatment of benign prostatic hyperplasia. Rev Urol 2006:8(Suppl 4):S3–9; with permission.)

Table 2
Doxazosin adverse effects

Adverse Effect	Doxazosin (%) (n = 665)	Placebo (%) (n = 300)
Dizziness (includes vertigo)	15.6[a]	9.0
Fatigue	8.0[a]	1.7
Hypotension	1.7[a]	0
Edema	2.7[a]	0.7
Dyspnea	2.6[a]	0.3

[a] $P \leq .05$ versus placebo.
From Lepor H. The evolution of alpha-blockers for the treatment of benign prostatic hyperplasia. Rev Urol 2006:8(Suppl 4):S53–9; with permission.

placebo at relieving symptoms and increasing PFRs (**Fig. 3**). Although the study was not powered to show differences between the 4- and 8-mg doses, in one of the pivotal trials the 8-mg dose was significantly superior to the 4-mg dose for improving LUTS. The adverse events attributable to tamsulosin were dose dependent and included dizziness, asthenia, and ejaculatory dysfunction. The incidences of ejaculatory dysfunction for placebo, 4 mg, and 8 mg tamsulosin were 0.2%, 8.4%, and 18.1%, respectively (**Table 3**). Interestingly, ejaculatory dysfunction was not previously observed with terazosin or doxazosin. Initially the pathophysiology of ejaculatory dysfunction was attributed to retrograde ejaculation due to alpha 1 blockade of bladder neck smooth muscle. Wolters and Hellstron[18] demonstrated that the tamsulosin ejaculatory dysfunction was anejaculation due to alpha-mediated inhibition of vassal and seminal vesicle smooth muscle.

A long-term open-label extension study demonstrated both the durability of response and the emergence of no safety issues.[19]

The advantage of tamsulosin over terazosin and doxazosin was the ability to administer a therapeutic dose without requirement for dose titration and the lack of postural hypotension. Initially, the pharmacologic property of tamsulosin that eliminated the requirement for dose titration was its presumed alpha 1a subtype selectivity. However, the binding and functional studies demonstrated that tamsulosin exhibited only a 10-fold selectivity for the alpha 1a versus alpha 1b subtypes and no alpha 1a versus alpha 1d selectivity.[20] This level of selectivity is likely not clinically relevant. In retrospect, the pharmacologic advantage of eliminating titration to an effective dose was explained by the slow-release formulation and not its negligible alpha 1 subtype selectivity.

There are several reasons why only the 4-mg dose was marketed for BPH. The manufacturers were able to claim that tamsulosin was the only alpha 1 blocker achieving a therapeutic response without dose titration. In addition, it was not feasible to manufacture an 8-mg single dose. There also seemed to be a significant dose response related to adverse events. Despite the high rates of ejaculatory dysfunction even at the 4-mg dose, tamsulosin became the market leader most likely because of the lack of dose titration and because generic terazosin and doxazosin were commercially available and the branded

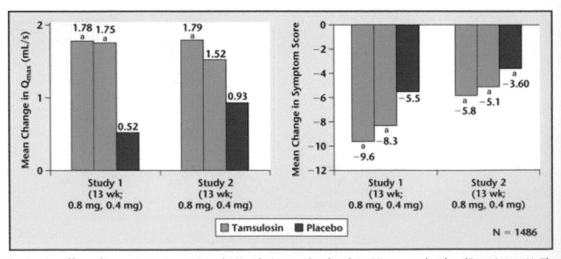

Fig. 3. The effect of tamsulosin on LUTS and PFR relative to placebo. [a] $P \leq .05$ versus placebo. (*From* Lepor H. The evolution of alpha-blockers for the treatment of benign prostatic hyperplasia. Rev Urol 2006:8(Suppl 4):53–9; with permission.)

Table 3
Tamsulosin adverse effects

Adverse Effect	Tamsulosin 0.4 mg (%) (n = 502)	Tamsulosin 0.8 mg (%) (n = 492)	Placebo (%) (n = 493)
Dizziness	14.9	17.1	10.1
Abnormal ejaculation	8.4	18.1	0.2
Asthenia	7.8	8.5	5.5
Libido decreased	1.0	2.0	1.2
Amblyopia	0.2	2.0	0.4

From Lepor H. The evolution of alpha-blockers for the treatment of benign prostatic hyperplasia. Rev Urol 2006:8(Suppl 4):S53–9; with permission.

drugs were no longer aggressively promoted by the industry.

The initial formulation of alfuzosin approved in Europe required twice-daily dosing.[21] A slow-release formulation of alfuzosin (alfuzosin SR) was subsequently developed, which allowed for once-daily dosing without the requirement for titration to an effective dose. Alfuzosin SR was the last alpha 1 blocker approved by the FDA for the treatment of BPH based on 2 pivotal randomized placebo-controlled studies.[22,23] Despite the fact alfuzosin did not exhibit any alpha 1 subtype selectivity, it was marketed as a uro-selective drug because in vivo studies in the cat model suggested the drug was more potent for relieving prostate urethral pressures than altering blood pressure.[24] The mechanism of physiologic uro-selectivity was attributed to enhanced penetration of the drug into the prostate. Subsequent in vivo studies failed to show physiologic uro-selectivity in the canine model.[24] The two alfuzosin pivotal

trials demonstrated both efficacy (**Fig. 4**) and excellent tolerance (**Table 4**). The primary advantage of alfuzosin was the lack of ejaculatory dysfunction associated with tamsulosin and lower incidences of asthenia and dizziness associated with terazosin and doxazosin. Because of the absence of ejaculatory dysfunction, alfuzosin was positioned for men who would be bothered by anejaculation. A comparison of the efficacy from all the pivotal trials suggests that alfuzosin is the least effective of the alpha 1 blockers. The superior tolerability and inferior efficacy suggests the 10-mg dose was achieving a relatively low level of alpha 1 blockade.

ALPHA 1 SUBTYPE SELECTIVE ALPHA-BLOCKERS

In the mid 1990s, 3 subtypes of the alpha 1 adrenoceptor (alpha 1a, alpha 1b, and alpha 1d) were characterized based on binding and functional

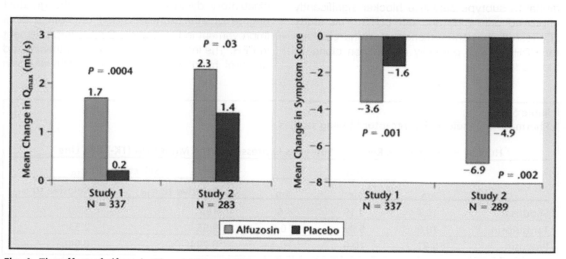

Fig. 4. The effect of alfuzosin SR on LUTS and PFR relative to placebo. Dosage: 10 mg/d. (*From* Lepor H. The evolution of alpha-blockers for the treatment of benign prostatic hyperplasia. Rev Urol 2006:8(Suppl 4):53–9; with permission.)

Table 4
Alfuzosin adverse effects

Adverse Effect	Alfuzosin (%) (n = 473)	Placebo (%) (n = 678)
Upper respiratory tract infection	3.0	0.6
Dizziness	5.7	2.8
Headache	3.0	1.8
Fatigue	2.7	1.8

From Lepor H. The evolution of alpha-blockers for the treatment of benign prostatic hyperplasia. Rev Urol 2006:8(Suppl 4):S53–9; with permission.

studies.[25,26] The alpha 1a subtype was dominant in the human prostate and was localized to the smooth muscle component of the prostate.[27,28] Prostate smooth muscle tension[29] and vascular smooth muscle tension[30] were mediated by the alpha 1a and alpha 1b subtypes, respectively. Based on the assumption that efficacy was mediated by alpha 1a subtype relaxation of prostate smooth muscle and the asthenia, dizziness, and postural hypotension were mediated by alpha 1b subtype relaxation of vascular smooth muscle, the race was on to develop an alpha 1a subtype selective antagonists for symptomatic BPH.

To the author's knowledge, Roche and Merck were the first pharmaceutical companies to cosponsor a randomized double-blind placebo-controlled proof-of-concept study evaluating the safety and efficacy of a highly selective alpha 1a blocker for the treatment of BPH. The outcome of the study was never published. The alpha 1a subtype selective blocker significantly improved only PFR and not LUTS. This study suggested that the efficacy of alpha-blockers for BPH did not primarily depend on alpha 1a blockade.

SILODOSIN, A UNIQUELY SELECTIVE ALPHA 1 SUBTYPE ANTAGONIST

The aforementioned experience with a highly selective alpha 1a blocker suggested that the cause of LUTS in men with BPH is not driven primarily by the alpha 1a subtype.

Subsequent studies demonstrated that the alpha 1d adrenoceptor is present in the bladder and nerve junctions.[31] Of all alpha-blockers commercially available, only silodosin exhibits clinically relevant degrees of alpha adrenoceptor subtype selectivity that can be leveraged in the clinical setting (**Tables 5** and **6**). Silodosin has been shown to exhibit a very high selectivity of alpha 1a versus alpha 1b adrenoceptors (162-fold selectivity), modest selectivity (55-fold selectivity) for alpha 1a versus alpha 1d adrenoceptors,[20] and 148-fold more potency for inhibiting alpha-mediated prostate versus mesenteric artery smooth muscle contraction (**Table 7**).[20,30,32] If efficacy is mediated by alpha 1a and alpha 1d adrenoceptors and toxicity by alpha 1b adrenoceptors, then silodosin has the potential for unique clinical properties.

Marks and colleagues[33] pooled the data from 2 pivotal trails performed in the United States evaluating the safety and efficacy of silodosin in men with LUTS BPH. In all 3 studies, the 8-mg daily dose of silodosin was administered without a dose titration. The efficacy (**Fig. 5**) and adverse events (see **Table 7**) of silodosin are summarized. Of all the alpha-blockers, the therapeutic effect on LUTS seems to be greatest with silodosin. The major limitation of silodosin is the high incidence of ejaculatory dysfunction. Roehrborn and colleagues[34] reported that those men experiencing ejaculatory dysfunction experience the greatest degree of effectiveness based on both a 30% improvement in LUTS and a 3 mL/s improvement in PFR. The incidence of dizziness, asthenia, and postural hypotension are on par with alfuzosin

Table 5
Pharmacologic selectivity: receptor binding studies

	Human α_1-Adrenergic Receptor Subtypes Expressed in the Mouse LM (TK-) Cell Line				
	pKi			Selectivity to α_{1A}	
	α_{1A}	α_{1B}	α_{1D}	Relative to α_{1B}	Relative to α_{1D}
Silodosin	10.4	8.19	8.66	162	55.0
Tamsulosin	10.9	9.92	10.5	9.55	2.51
Prazosin	9.91	10.6	10.1	0.204	0.646

Ratio expressed as the relative concentration.
From Lepor H. Pathophysiology of benign prostatic hyperplasia: insights from medical therapy for the disease. Rev Urol 2009:11(Suppl 1):S12; with permission.

Table 6
Uro-selectivity: inhibition of phenylephrine-mediated smooth muscle contraction

Compound	pA2*		α_{1A}/α_{1B}
	α_{1A}: Prostate	α_{1B}: Mesenteric Artery	
Silodosin	9.64 ± 0.12	7.47 ± 0.12	0.068
Prazosin	8.48 ± 0.04	9.15 ± 0.08	4.675
Tamsulosin	9.78 ± 0.09	9.36 ± 0.24	0.379

* negative logarithm of affinity to inhibit smooth muscle contraction.
From Lepor H. Pathophysiology of benign prostatic hyperplasia: insights from medical therapy for the disease. Rev Urol 2009:11(Suppl 1):S12; with permission.

and less than tamsulosin, terazosin, and doxazosin. The ability to maximize efficacy while minimizing adverse events with the exception of ejaculatory dysfunction without the requirement for dose titration is likely the result of silodosin's unique alpha 1 subtype selectivity.[35] Therefore, in the author's opinion, silodosin represents the best alpha-blocker for men with LUTS BPH providing ejaculatory dysfunction would be a tolerable adverse event. The only limitation of silodosin relative to other alpha-blockers in addition to the high incidence of ejaculatory dysfunction is that there is no commercially marketed generic; therefore, the cost versus benefits must be considered.

ALPHA-BLOCKERS FOR TREATING ACUTE URINARY RETENTION

Acute urinary retention (AUR) is a potentially life-threatening consequence of BPH. The initial management of AUR is to temporarily insert an indwelling urinary catheter. The catheter is typically removed in a few days in order to attempt a trial of voiding without a catheter. A randomized double-blind placebo-controlled study has shown that alfuzosin increases the likelihood of successfully removing the catheter while also decreasing the risk of a subsequent episode of AUR.[36] An episode of AUR is no longer an absolute indication for surgical intervention. Alpha-blockers are a very reasonable initial first-line option in the management of many episodes of AUR.

Table 7
Adverse events in silodosin registration trials

Adverse Event	Silodosin (%)	Placebo (%)
Anejaculation	28.1	0.9
Dizziness	3.2	1.1
Orthostatic hypotension	2.6	1.5
Nasal congestion	2.1	0.2

ALPHA-BLOCKERS VERSUS 5 ALPHA REDUCTASE INHIBITORS FOR TREATMENT OF LOWER URINARY TRACT SYMPTOMS/BENIGN PROSTATIC HYPERPLASIA

In the 1980s, the pathophysiology of LUTS BPH was attributed to BOO, which resulted in high-pressure, low-flow micturition and subsequent bladder dysfunction.[37] The cause for BOO was twofold: a dynamic component due to prostate smooth muscle tension and the static component due to the anatomic obstruction resulting from the enlarged prostate enlargement encroaching the bladder outlet. Therefore, medical therapies were targeted to relax prostate smooth muscle and reduce prostate volume using alpha-blockers and 5 alpha reductase inhibitors (5ARIs), respectively. Overall, approximately 80% and 20% of the hyperplastic volume is composed of stromal versus epithelial elements, respectively.[38–40] Half of the stromal hyperplasia is composed of smooth muscle elements.[39] Because 5ARIs promote only involution of prostatic epithelium, the observed reduction of prostate volume in response to these drugs is approximately 20%.[41,42] From only modest reduction of prostate volume, one would predict that the response to 5ARIs would be modest at best, especially in men without large prostate glands.

The relative effectiveness of 5ARIs and alpha-blockers was first investigated in the mid-1990s by the Veterans Affairs (VA) Cooperative Studies Benign Prostatic Hyperplasia Study Group.[43] A total of 1229 men with symptomatic BPH were randomized to receive terazosin, finasteride, the combination of terazosin and finasteride, or placebo for 1 year. The effectiveness of the treatment groups was captured by improvements in the American Urologic Association Symptom Score (AUASS) and PFR. The observed efficacy of terazosin in the VA study was similar to previous reports, whereas the effectiveness of finasteride was observed to be no greater than placebo (**Fig. 6**). Combination therapy was observed to be no

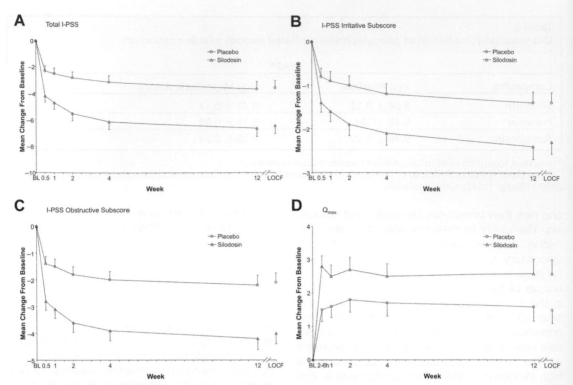

Fig. 5. Mean changes from baseline (BL) in total International Prostate Symptom Score (I-PSS) (A), I-PSS irritative subscore (B), I-PSS obstructive subscore (C), and Q_{max} (D). Earliest postdose I-PSS measurements occurred at week 0.5, and earliest postdose Q_{max} measurements occurred 2 to 6 hours after initial dosing. At all times differences between silodosin and placebo were statistically significant for total I-PSS ($P<.0001$), irritative subscore ($P<.001$), obstructive subscore ($P<.0001$), and Q_{max} ($P<.005$). Error bars indicate 95% confidence intervals. Measurements were based on observed cases except where indicated. LOCF, last observation carried forward. (*From* Marks LS, Gittelman MC, Hill LA, et al. Rapid efficacy of the highly selective alpha 1A-adrenoceptor antagonist silodosin in men with signs and symptoms of benign prostatic hyperplasia; pooled results of 2 phase 3 studies. J Urol 2009;181:2634; with permission.)

more effective than terazosin monotherapy because finasteride was of no clinical benefit relative to placebo. The primary difference between the study design of the VA trial and the finasteride registration studies was that the VA study enrolled all men with BPH, whereas the finasteride registration studies enrolled a disproportionate percentage of men with very large prostates, the subset most likely to respond to a drug whose mechanism of action is to reduce prostate size. Specifically, the mean prostate volume in the VA trial was 37 cm³ compared with 58.6 cm³ in the finasteride registration study. Therefore, the findings of the VA study reflect the effectiveness of medical therapies for all men with clinical BPH, whereas the findings of the finasteride registration study are relevant only to the subset of men with clinical BPH and very large prostates.

The effectiveness of terazosin and finasteride relative to placebo in the VA trial was subsequently examined according to baseline prostate volume.[44] Specifically, the efficacy of terazosin and

finasteride was examined for men with baseline prostate volumes less than 40 cm³ versus greater than 40 cm³. The efficacy of terazosin was independent of baseline prostate volume. In men with prostate volume less than 40 cm³, finasteride was equivalent to placebo. However, in men with prostate volumes greater than 40 cm³, the treatment-related effectiveness of finasteride relative to placebo for improvement in AUASS and PFR was 1.0 symptom unit and 1.6 mL/s, respectively. The magnitude of treatment-related efficacy observed in the larger prostates (>40 cm³) receiving finasteride is similar to the treatment-related efficacy in the finasteride registration studies.[41,42] In larger prostates, terazosin was more effective than finasteride at improving LUTS.

The findings of the VA study were replicated by the Prospective European Doxazosin and Combination Therapy Study (PREDICT),[45] which substituted the alpha-blocker doxazosin for terazosin. Doxazosin was significantly more effective than placebo at relieving LUTS and increasing

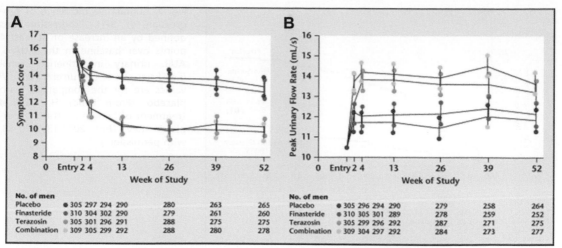

Fig. 6. Comparison of finasteride, terazosin, and combined dosing regimens for the treatment of BPH. Symptom scores and flow rates are expressed as adjusted means and 95% confidence intervals. (*A*) AUASS, according to treatment group. Symptom scores of subjects who received terazosin or combination therapy were significantly lower from baseline, as well as from those in the placebo and finasteride groups, at all follow-up visits. (*B*) Mean peak urinary flow rates were significantly higher in the terazosin and combination therapy groups than in the placebo and finasteride groups at all follow-up visits. (*From* Lepor H. Medical treatment of benign prostatic hyperplasia. Rev Urol 2011;13(1):24; with permission.)

PFR, and finasteride was no more effective than placebo; there was no benefit of combination therapy over alpha-blocker monotherapy. In PREDICT, the baseline prostate volume was 36 cm³, which is virtually identical to the VA study.

The VA and PREDICT studies were designed to examine the relative effectiveness of alpha-blockers, 5ARIs, and the combination of these two drugs for improving LUTS and BOO. The Medical Therapy of Prostatic Symptoms (MTOPS) study was designed to address the ability of medical therapy to alter disease progression.[46] MTOPS examined the ability of a 5ARI (finasteride), an alpha-blocker (doxazosin), and combination therapy (finasteride + doxazosin) to prevent disease progression relative to placebo. In this randomized, multicenter, placebo-controlled study enrolling 3047 men with clinical BPH, the primary end point was clinical BPH progression. Clinical BPH progression was defined as a 4-point increase in International Prostate Symptom Score or development of AUR, renal insufficiency, urinary tract infection (UTI), or incontinence. The requirement for invasive therapy due to BPH was not included in the definition of disease progression but was captured independently. With a mean follow-up of 4.5 years, all treatment groups significantly decreased overall disease progression relative to placebo (**Fig. 7**). Combination therapy was significantly more effective than the monotherapies at preventing overall disease progression. In the placebo group, 80% and 15% of the

events contributing to overall clinical progression were attributable to symptom progression and the development of AUR, respectively. Doxazosin and finasteride were equally effective at preventing LUTS progression, whereas finasteride was significantly more effective than doxazosin at preventing AUR. Although the risk reduction rate for preventing AUR in the combination group relative to placebo was 81%, only 18 men developed AUR in the placebo group. Overall, 786 men were treated with combination therapy over a mean follow-up of 4.5 years to prevent 61, 14, and 25 symptom progression events, episodes of AUR, and invasive therapies for BPH, respectively. This finding translates into a need to treat 12, 56, and 29 men with clinical BPH for a mean of 4.5 years to prevent a single man from developing symptom progression, AUR, or invasive therapy for BPH.

In summary, alpha-blockers represent the drug of choice for improving LUTS independent of prostate volume. For those men with bothersome LUTS and large prostates who have some symptom response to terazosin, adding a 5ARI is a reasonable option. Men with large prostates are at greatest risk for developing AUR, and a 5ARI is the most effective strategy to prevent AUR in men with large glands. Combination therapy is a reasonable first-line treatment in men with large prostates whereby the clinical indication is to both relieve LUTS and decrease the risk of AUR.

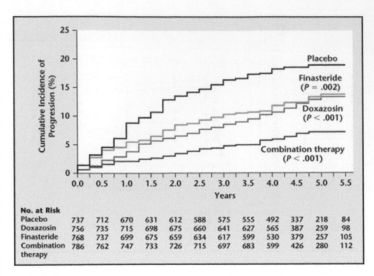

Fig. 7. Cumulative incidence of progression of BPH. Progression was defined by an increase of at least 4 points over baseline in the AUASS, AUR, urinary incontinence, renal insufficiency, or recurrent UTI. *P* values are for the comparison with placebo. (*From* Lepor H. Medical treatment of benign prostatic hyperplasia. Rev Urol 2011;13(1):20–33; with permission.)

WHAT IS THE MECHANISM FOR ALPHA 1 BLOCKERS IN THE TREATMENT OF BENIGN PROSTATIC HYPERPLASIA?

In the mid 1980s, the author was convinced that alpha-blockers relieved LUTS by decreasing BOO.[36] There is increasing evidence that this proposed mechanism of efficacy for alpha-blockers in men with LUTS/BPH is an oversimplification.

In order to prove that the mechanism of alpha-blockers was medicated by smooth muscle relaxation, Shapiro and colleagues[47] biopsied the prostates of 26 men before initiating alpha-blocker therapy. The percent of smooth muscle in the prostate biopsies was quantified, and the improvement in baseline AUASS and PFR following treatment with terazosin was ascertained. The improvement in PFR was highly correlated with the amount of prostate smooth muscle, whereas improvement in LUTS was not correlated with the amount of smooth muscle. This study was initially designed to confirm that the mechanism of alpha-blocker mediated improvement in LUTS was mediated by prostate smooth muscle. However at conclusion the findings suggested the contrary.

A review of the VA Cooperative Study of Medical Therapy for BPH demonstrated that there was at best a very weak correlation between improvement in LUTS (change in AUASS) and BOO (improvement in uroflow) in the terazosin-treated group.[44] Interestingly, the lack of correlation between change in AUASS and BOO was also observed in men undergoing transurethral resection of the prostate (TURP).[48] If alpha-blockers and TURP relieve LUTS by decreasing BOO, then a strong correlation should have been

observed between these end points. This analysis suggested that TURP and alpha-blockers relieve both LUTS and BOO but through divergent mechanisms.

All of the medical therapy BPH studies enrolled men with low baseline PFR to ensure medical therapy was being offered to men with BOO. If the pathophysiology of BPH/LUTS is due to BOO, it would be unreasonable to enroll men into a medical therapy for a BPH trial who did not have BOO. One would then anticipate that those men with the greatest degree of BOO should experience the greatest symptom improvement. However, men in the lowest quartile baseline PFR in the VA trial (5.0–8.6 mL/s) experienced the same level of LUTS improvement as those in the highest quartile baseline PFR (12.4–15.0 mL/s).[43] This finding prompted a study examining the effect of terazosin on men with LUTS/BPH independent of baseline PFR.[49] The change in LUTS was similar in men with a PFR less than 15 mL/s and a PFR greater than 15 mL/s, indicating that men with and without baseline BOO achieve similar levels of symptom improvement with alpha-blockers. Not surprisingly, those men with normal baseline PFRs did not experience an increase in their PFRs on terazosin.

The author and colleagues also examined the VA Cooperative Study to gain insights on the mechanism for adverse events attributed to alpha-blocker.[50] It was presumed that asthenia and dizziness were due to vascular mediated events. The author and colleagues were unable to identify a correlation between blood pressure changes and these adverse events suggesting that asthenia and dizziness may be centrally medicated.

Other clinical studies have shown a disassociation between changes in LUTS and PFR. As discussed earlier, a highly selective alpha 1a subtype antagonist improved PFR without improving LUTS. In addition, phosphodiesterase inhibitors have been shown to improve LUTS in men with LUTS/BPH without any increase in BOO.[51,52]

ALPHA-BLOCKERS AS THE TREATMENT OF BENIGN PROSTATIC HYPERPLASIA IN THE YEAR 2016

Alpha-blockers were approved for the indication of BPH 24 years ago. Today, this class of drugs remains the first-line treatment of LUTS/BPH. The evolution of alpha-blockers has been to eliminate the requirement for dose titration and improve tolerability while preserving efficacy. Silodosin is the most recently FDA-approved alpha-blocker for BPH/LUTS. Silodosin has significantly reduced adverse events, such as asthenia and dizziness, at the expense of ejaculatory dysfunction.[35] If ejaculatory dysfunction proves to be a bothersome adverse event, then alfuzosin represents a reasonable second option realizing efficacy likely will be somewhat compromised.

Several other drugs, such as phosphodiesterase (PDE) 5 inhibitors,[51,52] anticholinergic drugs,[52] and beta agonists,[53,54] have been shown to improve LUTS in men. For virtually all men in whom the goal is to relieve LUTS/BPH, an alpha-blocker remains the best first option. In those men who exhibit some response to an alpha-blocker but remain bothered by their LUTS, it is reasonable to add a PDE 5 inhibitor, an anticholinergic agent, or a 5ARI if there is evidence of coexisting erectile dysfunction, a large prostate, or a small bladder and overactive bladder, respectively.

REFERENCES

1. Caine M, Raz S, Zeigler M. Adrenergic and cholinergic receptors in the human prostate, prostatic capsule and bladder neck. Br J Urol 1975;27: 193–202.
2. Caine M, Pfau A, Perlberg S. The use of alpha adrenergic blockers in benign prostatic obstruction. Br J Urol 1976;48:255–63.
3. Caine M, Perlberg S, Meretyk S. A placebo-controlled double-blind study of the effect of phenoxybenzamine in benign prostatic obstruction. Br J Urol 1978;50:551–4.
4. Lepor H, Shapiro E. Characterization of the alpha₁ adrenergic receptor in human benign prostatic hyperplasia. J Urol 1984;132:1226.
5. Shapiro E, Lepor H. Alpha₂ adrenergic receptors in hyperplastic human prostate: identification and characterization using [3h] rauwolscine. J Urol 1986;135:1038.
6. Lepor H, Gup DI, Baumann M, et al. Laboratory assessment of terazosin and alpha₁ blockade in prostatic hyperplasia. Urology 1988;32(6):21.
7. Kirby RS, Coppinger SWC, Corcoran MO, et al. Prazosin in the treatment prostatic obstruction: a placebo-controlled study. Br J Urol 1987;60:136–42.
8. Lepor H, Auerbach S, Puras-Baez A, et al. A multicenter fixed-dose study of the safety and efficacy of terazosin in the treatment of the symptoms of benign prostatic hyperplasia. J Urol 1992;148: 1467–74.
9. Brawer MK, Adams G, Epstein H, et al. Terazosin in the treatment of benign prostatic hyperplasia. Arch Fam Med 1993;2:929–35.
10. Lloyd SN, Buckley JF, Chilton CP, et al. Terazosin in the treatment of benign prostatic hyperplasia: a multi-center, placebo-controlled trial. Br J Urol 1992;70(Suppl 1):17–21.
11. Lepor H, the Terazosin Research Group. Long-term efficacy and safety of terazosin in patients with benign prostatic hyperplasia. Urology 1995;45: 406–13.
12. Fawzy A, Braun K, Lewis GP, et al. Doxazosin in the treatment of benign prostatic hyperplasia in normotensive patients: a multicenter study. J Urol 1995; 154:105–9.
13. Gillenwater JY, Corm RL, Chrysant SG, et al. Doxazosin for the treatment of benign prostatic hyperplasia in patients with mild to moderate essential hypertension: a double-blind, placebo-controlled dose response multicenter study. J Urol 1995;154: 110–5.
14. Lepor H, Kaplan SA, Klimberg I, et al. Doxazosin in benign prostatic hyperplasia: long-term efficacy and safety in hypertensive and normotensive patients. J Urol 1997;157:525–30.
15. MacDiarmid SA, Emery RT, Ferguson SF, et al. A randomized double-blind study assessing 4 versus 8 mg doxazosin for benign prostatic hyperplasia. J Urol 1999;162:1629–32.
16. Lepor H, the Tamsulosin Investigator Group. Phase III multicenter, placebo-controlled study of tamsulosin in benign prostatic hyperplasia. Urology 1998; 51:892–900.
17. Naayan P, Tewari A, the United States 93-01 Study Group. A second phase III multicenter placebo controlled study of 2 dosages of modified release tamsulosin in patients with symptoms of benign prostatic hyperplasia. J Urol 1998;160: 1701–6.
18. Wolters JP, Hellstrom WJG. Current concepts in ejaculatory dysfunction. Rev Urol 2006;8(Suppl 4): 518–25.

19. Lepor H, the Tamsulosin Investigator Group. Long-term evaluation of tamsulosin in benign prostatic hyperplasia: phase III extension. Urology 1998;51: 901–6.

20. Tatemichi S, Kobayashi K, Maezawa A, et al. Alpha1-adrenoceptor subtype selectivity and organ specificity of silodosin (KMD-3213). Yakugaku Zasshi 2006;126:209–16.

21. Jardin A, Bensadoun H, Delauche-Cavallier MC, et al. Alfuzosin for treatment of benign prostatic hypertrophy. Lancet 1991;337:1457–61.

22. Van Kerrebroeck P, Jardin A, Laval ZKU, et al. Efficacy and safety of new prolonged release formulation of patients with symptomatic benign prostatic hyperplasia. Eur Urol 2000;37:306–13.

23. Roehrborn CG, for the AFFUS Study Group. Efficacy and safety on once-daily alfuzosin in the treatment of lower urinary tract symptoms and clinical benign prostatic hyperplasia: a randomized placebo-controlled trial. Urology 2001;58:953–9.

24. Lefvre-Borg F, O'Connor SE, Schoemaker H, et al. Alfuzosin, a selective alpha-1 adrenoceptor antagonist in the lower urinary tract. Br J Pharmacol 1993; 109:1282–9.

25. Kenny BA, Naylor AM, Carter AJ, et al. Effect of alpha1 adrenoceptor antagonists on prostatic pressure and blood pressure in the anesthetized dog. Urology 1994;44:52–7.

26. Michel MC, Kenny B, Schwinn DA. Classification of α-adrenoceptors. Naunyn Schmiedebergs Arch Pharmacol 1995;352:1–10.

27. Lepor H, Tang R, Kobayashi S, et al. Localization of the alpha$_{1a}$ adrenoceptor in the human prostate. J Urol 1995;154:2096–9.

28. Lepor H, Zhang W, Kobayashi S, et al. A comparison of the binding and functional properties of alpha$_1$ adrenoceptors and smooth muscle content of the human, canine and rat prostate. J Pharmacol Exp Ther 1994;270:722–7.

29. Forray C, Bard JA, Wetzel JM, et al. The alpha$_1$ adrenergic receptor that mediates smooth muscle contraction in human prostate has pharmacologic properties of the cloned human alpha$_{1c}$ subtype. Mol Pharm 1994;45:703–8.

30. Murata S, Taniguchi T, Takahashi M, et al. Tissue selectivity of KMD-3213, an α$_1$-adrenoceptor antagonist in human prostate and vasculature. J Urol 2000;164:578–83.

31. Schwinn DA, Roehrborn CG. Alpha 1-adrenoceptor subtypes and lower urinary tract symptoms. Int J Urol 2008;15:193–9.

32. Lepor H. Medical treatment of benign prostatic hyperplasia. Rev Urol 2011;13(1):20–3.

33. Marks LS, Gittelman MC, Hill LA, et al. Rapid efficacy of the highly selective alpha 1A-adrenoceptor antagonist silodosin in men with signs and symptoms of benign prostatic hyperplasia: pooled results of 2 phase 3 studies. J Urol 2009;181:2634.

34. Roehrborn CG, Kaplan SA, Lepor H, et al. Symptomatic and urodynamic responses in patients with reduced or no seminal emission during silodosin treatment for LUTS and BPH. Prostate Cancer Prostatic Dis 2011;14(2):143–8.

35. Lepor H, Hill LA. Silodosin for the treatment of benign prostatic hyperplasia: pharmacology and cardiovascular tolerability. Pharmacotherapy 2010; 30:1303–12.

36. McNeil SA, Daruwala PD, Mitchell ID, et al. Sustained-release alfuzosin and trial without catheter after acute urinary retention: a prospective placebo-controlled. BJU Int 1999;84:622–7.

37. Lepor H. Nonsurgical management of benign prostatic hyperplasia. J Urol 1989;141:1283–9.

38. Barsch G, Muller HR, Oberholzer M, et al. Light microscopic stereological analysis of the normal human prostate and of benign prostatic hyperplasia. J Urol 1979;122:487–9.

39. Shapiro E, Becich MJ, Lepor H. The relative proportion of stromal and epithelial hyperplasia as related to the development of clinical BPH. J Urol 1992; 147:1293–7.

40. Shapiro E, Hartanto V, Lepor H. Quantifying the smooth muscle content of the prostate using double-immunoenzymatic staining and color assisted image analysis. J Urol 1992;147:1167–70.

41. Gormley GJ, Stoner E, Bruskewitz RC, et al. The effect of finasteride in men with benign prostatic hyperplasia. N Engl J Med 1992;327:1185–91.

42. Finasteride (MK-906) in the treatment of benign prostatic hyperplasia. The Finasteride Study Group. Prostate 1993;22:291–9.

43. Lepor H, Williford WO, Barry MJ, et al. The efficacy of terazosin, finasteride, or both in benign prostatic hyperplasia. N Engl J Med 1996;335:533–9.

44. Lepor H, Williford WO, Barry MJ. The impact of medical therapy on bother due to symptoms, quality of life and global outcome and factors predicting response of medical therapy: an analysis of the VA study of BPH. J Urol 1998;160:1358–67.

45. Kirby RS, Roehrborn C, Boyle P, et al, for the Prospective European Doxazosin and Combination Therapy Study Investigators. Efficacy and tolerability of doxazosin and finasteride, alone or in combination, in treatment of symptomatic benign prostatic hyperplasia: the prospective European doxazosin and combination therapy (PREDICT) trial. Urol 2003;61:119–26.

46. McConnell JD, Andriole GL Jr, Bautista O, et al. The long-term effects of doxazosin, finasteride and the combination on the clinical progression of benign prostatic hyperplasia. N Engl J Med 2003;349:25.

47. Shapiro E, Hartanto V, Lepor H. The response to alpha blockade in benign prostatic hyperplasia is

related to the percent area density of prostate smooth muscle. Prostate 1992;21:297–307.

48. Lepor H, Rigaud G. The efficacy of transurethral resection of the prostate in men with moderate symptoms of prostatism. J Urol 1990;143:533–7.

49. Lepor H, Nieder A, Dixon CM, et al. The effectiveness of terazosin in men with normal and abnormal peak flow rates. Urology 1997;49:476–80.

50. Lepor H, Jones K, Williford W. The mechanism of adverse events associated with terazosin: an analysis of the Veteran's Affairs cooperative study. J Urol 2000;163(4):1134–7.

51. McVary KT, Monnig W, Camps JL Jr, et al. Sildenafil citrate improves erectile function and urinary symptoms in men with erectile dysfunction and lower urinary tract symptoms associated with benign prostatic hyperplasia: a randomized, double-blind trial. Urology 2007;177:1071–7.

52. McVary KT, Roehrborn CG, Kaminetsky JC, et al. Tadalafil relieves lower urinary tract symptoms secondary to benign prostatic hyperplasia. Urology 2007; 177:1401–7.

53. Füllhase C, Chapple C, Cornu JN, et al. Systematic review of combination drug therapy for non-neurogenic male lower urinary tract symptoms. Eur Urol 2013;64:228–43.

54. Ogura K, Sengiku A, Miyazaki Y, et al. Effects of add-on mirabegron on storage symptoms in men with lower urinary tract symptoms receiving alpha-1 blocker therapy. Eur Urol 2013;(Suppl 12e):1091.

5-Alpha-Reductase Inhibitors and Combination Therapy

Claudius Füllhase, MD, PhD[a],*, Marc P. Schneider, MD[b]

KEYWORDS

- 5-Alpha-reductase inhibitors • Finasteride • Dutasteride • Combination drug therapy
- Prostatic hyperplasia • Lower urinary tract symptoms

KEY POINTS

- In men suffering from benign prostatic hyperplasia (BPH) with lower urinary tract symptoms (LUTS), 5-alpha reductase inhibitors (5ARIs) are a treatment option when prostate size is greater than 30 to 40 mL and medical treatment is intended for longer than 1 year.
- In the same patients, combination of 5ARIs with alpha-adrenergic-blockers (ABs) is a better option in regard to symptomatic improvement and reduction of disease progression if they are suitable for potential AB-related side effects.
- Potential sexual side effects of 5ARIs and 5ARI/AB combinations might be an individual exclusion criterion and should be openly discussed with each patient.
- 5ARIs are not recommended for the prevention of BPH/LUTS or prostate cancer (PCa). Patients with BPH/LUTS undergoing 5ARI therapy should be routinely screened for PCa, at which time the serum prostate-specific antigen level should be doubled.
- Combination of phosphodiesterase type 5 inhibitors with 5ARIs might be the best medical treatment option for some patients; however, more clinical evidence is needed.

INTRODUCTION

5-Alpha-reductases (5ARs) are enzymes converting testosterone into dihydrotestosterone (DHT).[1] DHT is the most important hormone for the development and function of male sex organs.[2] Genetic defects of 5ARs can result in pseudohermaphroditism, meaning a female phenotype despite the presence of XY genotype.[3] In 1940, Charles Huggins first reported the relationship between testosterone and benign prostatic hyperplasia (BPH) development.[4] In the 1970s, the crucial role of 5AR-depending testosterone to DHT transformation in BPH development became apparent by the seminal works of Jean Wilson.[5,6] Realizing the therapeutic potential of DHT regulation

resulted in a quest for an 5AR-inhibitor (5ARI), which ended in 1992 with the approval of finasteride (FIN; Proscar) by the US Food and Drug Administration (FDA).[7] In 2002, the FDA approved dutasteride (DUT; Avodart) as another 5ARI.[7] According to current guidelines, both 5ARIs can be used in the treatment of BPH with lower urinary tract symptoms (LUTS), either alone or in combination with other drugs targeting BPH/LUTS.[8,9]

5-ALPHA-REDUCTASE INHIBITOR MONOTHERAPY
Finasteride

After several animal experiments, MK-906 (which later became FIN) was successfully tested for

Disclosures: Nothing to disclose.
[a] Department of Urology, University of Rostock, Ernst-Heydemann-Str. 6, Rostock 18057, Germany; [b] Department of Health Science and Technology, Swiss Federal Institute of Technology Zurich, Brain Research Institute, University of Zurich, Winterthurerstrasse 190, Zürich 8057, Switzerland
* Corresponding author.
E-mail address: Claudius.fuellhase@uni-rostock.de

safety, tolerability, and biochemical activity in 350 volunteers.[10] In healthy men, MK-906 reduced serum DHT levels by −62% to −82% without affecting serum testosterone levels.[11,12] Intraprostatic DHT levels were reduced by −92% in men awaiting prostate surgery.[13]

In a phase III clinical trial, 895 men with BPH received either placebo (PBO) or FIN 1 to 5 mg for 1 year.[14] The Boyarski score (a precursor of the American Urological Association symptom score [AUA-SS] or the international prostate symptom score [IPSS]) was significantly reduced by −2.7 with 5 mg FIN compared with no changes with PBO and 1 mg FIN.[14] The urinary flow rate (Q_{max}) significantly increased from 5.6 to 6.4 mL/s with 5 mg FIN and from 5.3 to 6.1 mL/s with 1 mg FIN but remained at baseline with PBO (5.6 and 5.8 mL/s).[14] Prostate size was reduced by −19% compared with baseline with 5 mg FIN, by −18% with 1 mg FIN, and insignificantly by −3% with PBO.[14] In an open-label extension 186 men continued to take 5 mg FIN for 4 more years.[15] Prostate volume reached a nadir at 24 months (−24% of initial size) and was maintained for the rest of the study. Similarly the symptom score improvement of −4.3 points and the increase of Q_{max} by 2.3 mL/s were maintained for 4 years.[15]

In another trial, 3040 men with BPH received either FIN 5 mg or PBO for 4 years.[16] AUA-SS was reduced by −3.3 with FIN and by −1.3 with PBO. Prostate volume was reduced by −18% with FIN and increased by 14% with PBO. Q_{max} improved by 1.9 mL/s with FIN and remained at 0.2 mL/s with PBO.[16] However, the most remarkable findings were a −57% risk reduction of acute urinary retention (AUR) and a −55% risk reduction to undergo prostate surgery when taking FIN.[16] This effect was confirmed and sustained in an open-label extension, in which 908 subjects took part for another 2 years.[17] Subjects who switched from PBO to FIN during extension showed at study end the same AUR reduction and prostate surgery incidence as the continuous FIN arm.[17]

Various other clinical trials compared FIN 5 mg versus PBO and reported similar outcomes, which means a reduction of prostate size by −15% to −21%, an IPSS (or similar score) reduction by −13% to −38%, and an increase of Q_{max} by 1.6 to 2.2 mL/s.[18–22] In all studies, these effects were measurable after 6 to 12 months. Meta-analysis revealed that the difference in improvement between FIN and PBO becomes significant when the prostate volume is greater than 40 mL at baseline.[23] According to a Cochrane systematic database review, the symptomatic improvements of FIN occur distinctly later than the effects of alpha-blockers (ABs).[24] However, when taken

longer than 1 year, FIN reduces BPH progression and the risk to undergo prostate surgery, which is not an effect of ABs.[24]

Summing up all evidence, and according to current guideline recommendations, FIN monotherapy is a treatment option in men with moderate to severe LUTS and an enlarged prostate (>40 mL).[8,9] FIN should not be used in men with LUTS without prostatic enlargement.[8] Furthermore, FIN can be used to prevent disease progression in regard to AUR and the need for surgery.[8,9] Due to the low onset of action, FIN is only suitable for long-term treatment.[9]

Dutasteride

In a study, 4325 men with clinical BPH received either DUT 0.5 mg or PBO over a 2 year period. At study end, serum DHT was reduced by −92%, prostate size by −25%, AUA SS by −4.5 points, and Q_{max} was increased by 2.2 mL/s with DUT.[25] Risk reduction for AUR was −57%, and −48% for prostatic surgery compared with PBO.[25] In an open-label extension, 1570 subjects were enrolled. After 2 more years, prostate size was reduced by −26%, AUA-SS by −6.1, and Q_{max} increased by 2.8 mL/s with DUT.[26] The values for subjects, who switched from PBO to DUT were −20% prostate size, −5.3 AUA-SS, and +1.8 mL/s Q_{max}.[26] The effects of DUT were faster and more pronounced the greater the prostate volume was at baseline.[27] In a post hoc analysis of the Reduction by DUT of Prostate Cancer Events (REDUCE) study, 1617 men with a prostate greater than 40 mL were evaluated.[28] Clinical progression, as defined by either AUR, need for prostatic surgery, or symptom deterioration defined by an IPSS increase greater than 4, occurred in 36% of PBO and 21% of DUT subjects, translating into an absolute risk reduction by −15% and a relative risk reduction of −41%.[28]

Whereas FIN inhibits the 5AR isoform type II, DUT inhibits 5AR isoform type I and type II; therefore it is called a dual inhibitor. Post hoc analysis suggests that the effects of DUT, in contrast to FIN, are also significant in subjects with a prostate size between 30 to 40 mL.[29] However, different inclusion criteria in the clinical trials evaluating FIN and DUT make it difficult to directly compare these 5ARIs. The Enlarged Prostate International Comparator Study (EPICS) was designed to evaluate differences between DUT and FIN.[30] In this trial, 1630 men with BPH received either DUT 0.5 mg or FIN 5 mg for 1 year. There were no significant differences in regard to prostate size, AUA-SS reduction, Q_{max} improvement, or the timely onset of their effects.[30] Hence, the pharmacological differences between those 2 compounds are not represented by any meaningful clinical difference, at least in regard to BPH/LUTS treatment. Accordingly, the guideline recommendation for DUT is the same as that for FIN, which is a long-term therapeutic option in men with moderate to severe LUTS and an increased prostate size (>40 mL).[9]

Side Effects and Further Aspects of 5-Alpha-Reductase Inhibitors

Adverse side effects

Erectile dysfunction (ED), decreased libido, ejaculatory disorders (EjDs), and gynecomastia are the only adverse side effects that consistently occur significantly more often with 5ARIs than with PBO in various clinical trials. In a review evaluating studies ranging from 6 to 54 months, FIN increased episodes of ED by 15%, DUT by 11.0%, and PBO by 6%.[31] EjD increased by 7% with FIN, by 3% with DUT, and by 0.1% to 1% with PBO.[31] Decreased libido occurred 18% more often with FIN, by 6% with DUT, and by 3% to 6% with PBO.[31] In another retrospective analysis, however, FIN was reported to have fewer sexual side effects than DUT.[32] In 378 men treated for 5 years with 5ARIs, the incidence of ED, EjD, and decreased libido leading to discontinuation from therapy occurred in 2.1%, 1.8%, and 1.4% with FIN, and in 5.1%, 2.4%, and 2.7%, with DUT, respectively.[32] Additionally self-reported gynecomastia was reported in 3.5% with DUT and in 1.2% with FIN.[32] EPICS, which was the only trial directly comparing FIN versus DUT, reported no significant difference regarding any adverse side effect.[30] ED occurred in 8% to 9% with 5ARI, decreased libido in 5% to 6%, EjD in 2%, and gynecomastia in 1%.[30] Drug-related adverse events (AEs) leading to study withdrawal occurred in 3% of 5ARI treated subjects during 2 years.[30] The Proscar Long-term Efficacy and Safety Study (PLESS) reported that men treated with FIN experience sexual side effects within the first year of drug treatment but not thereafter.[33] Similarly, it was reported for DUT that the incidence of sexual AEs decreased with longer therapy duration.[34] Even though side effects of 5ARIs are generally considered to be mild, the possibility of sexual side effects should be openly discussed with a patient before commencing therapy.[31]

Due to their good tolerability and safety, 5ARIs are considered suitable or beneficial drugs for older patients and frail elderly people according to the Fit For Age (FORTA) classification.[35] 5ARI were reported to not negatively affect bone mineral density, serum lipoprotein, or hemoglobin levels.[36] Neither FIN nor DUT were reported to increase bone fracture risk.[37] In older hypogonadal men suffering from musculoskeletal negative effects of testosterone deficiency (serum testosterone concentration <300 ng/dL), testosterone replacement therapy (125 mg/wk) could be successfully coadministered with FIN 5 mg.[38] After 1 year of combined treatment, subjects showed increased muscle strength and bone mineral density, with simultaneously increased serum testosterone levels and still lowered serum DHT levels, compared with PBO or FIN alone.[38] Prostate size significantly increased by 5.3 mL in the testosterone group, decreased by −5.7 mL with FIN, and stayed at baseline with testosterone/FIN and with PBO alone.[38] FIN alone did not affect muscle strength or bone mineral density.[38] However, the study included only 60 subjects.[38] Another very small study reported significant prostate size reduction by DUT in men with an ongoing testosterone replacement therapy.[39] Evidence is too scarce to give recommendations; however, testosterone replacement therapy with simultaneous 5ARI therapy might be a therapeutic option in selected patients undergoing close-meshed follow-up. The effects of testosterone/5ARI combination on prostate cancer risk are not known.

Further aspects

Additionally to its use in the treatment of BPH/LUTS, FIN is approved and used for the treatment of androgenetic alopecia.[40] For this indication, FIN is available in a 1 mg formulation (Propecia), which is not recommended to be used for BPH/LUTS treatment.

5ARIs can affect prostatic bleeding. In small studies FIN was shown to reduce the risk of prostatic hematuria recurrence.[41,42] The AUA states in the guidelines that FIN is a treatment alternative in men with refractory hematuria due to prostatic bleeding after exclusion of any other cause.[8] This view is not shared with the European Association of Urology (EAU) guidelines. Similarly, FIN might be successfully used in the treatment of refractory hematospermia.[43] However, available literature is too scarce to give any recommendation. Some investigators report decreased intraoperative blood loss during transurethral resection of the prostate (TURP) and consequently reduced need for blood transfusions in patients undergoing 5ARI treatment.[44–46] Some investigators report that this blood-saving effect of 5ARIs could also be reached with a short-term (6–8 weeks) preoperative treatment.[47,48] However, this beneficial effect of 5ARI treatment seems to be restricted to patients with rather large prostates (>50 mL).[48] Also, 5ARI might make certain operations, such as laser enucleations, even more difficult to perform.[49] A recent meta-analysis, including 1489 subjects, stated that there was a significant reduction of blood loss per gram of resected prostate tissue in favor of 5ARIs; however, there was no significant reduction of blood transfusions or operative time with 5ARI compared with PBO or no treatment.[50] The AUA states that there is insufficient evidence to recommend 5ARIs preoperatively to TURP.[8]

Data from 9253 men without BPH/LUTS from the Prostate Cancer Prevention Trial (PCPT) suggest that FIN could have a role in the prevention of incident BPH because 18.6 per 1000 person-years in the PBO but only 11.2 per 1000 person-years in the FIN group developed incident BPH, defined as first event of medical or surgical treatment, or sustained BPH symptoms in the form of an IPSS greater than 14.[51] In other words, the number needed to treat (NNT) to prevent 1 case of clinical BPH over 7 years was 58 for men aged 55 to 59, 42 for men aged 60 to 64, and 31 for men 65 years and older.[51] However, due to the controversies regarding 5ARIs and prostate cancer risk, the use of 5ARIs in BPH prevention should be considered very carefully. Current guidelines make no statement about the use of 5ARIs in BPH prevention.[8,9]

Effects of 5-alpha-reductase inhibitors on prostate-specific antigen levels and prostate cancer risk

5ARIs are known to reduce serum prostate-specific antigen (PSA) levels and, as such, limit the value of serum PSA in PCa screening if not considered. The Finasteride PSA Study Group recommends doubling the measured serum PSA level in BPH patients taking 5ARIs so that a PCa diagnosis is not masked.[52] The same recommendation was given by the PLESS group and other investigators.[53,54] After 7 years of 5ARI treatment, serum PSA level should be corrected by the factor 2.5.[55]

Triggered by a surprising post hoc finding of the Combination of Avodart and Tamsulosin (CombAT) trial, in which subjects receiving DUT had a lower rate of positive prostate biopsies, a passionate discussion regarding the role of 5ARI in PCa prevention started and resulted in the initiation of 2 large trials: PCPT and REDUCE.[56,57] In these trials, 18,882 men older than 55 years without BPH received either FIN or PBO for 7 years.[56] During this period, PCa was reduced by almost −25% with FIN.[56] However, those desirable effects were counterweighed by the finding that the number of high-risk PCa was significantly higher in the FIN (37%) than in the PBO group (22%).[56] Similarly, REDUCE reported a −22%

risk reduction of PCa diagnosis with DUT.[57] At the same time the likelihood to get diagnosed with a high-risk PCa was significantly higher with DUT than with PBO.[57] Those controversial findings resulted in a debate about the pros and cons of 5ARI treatment in PCa prevention. To address this issue, the FDA performed an extensive work-up (including histological re-examination of specimen and various statistical calculations). Their final conclusion was that 5ARIs indeed increases the risk for high-grade PCa and excluded any bias or confounding factor.[58] The FDA summed up that there is no acceptable risk to benefit ratio; thus 5ARI cannot be recommended routinely for PCa prevention.[58]

The Health Professionals Follow-up Study includes a prospective cohort of 51,529 men since 1986.[59] Out of this cohort, 2878 men could be identified who had taken a 5ARI. At the same time, 3681 men were diagnosed with PCa and 289 had died from it. In this observational study, no correlation between high-risk or lethal PCa and 5ARI intake could be established.[59] Guidelines recommend that men taking 5ARIs for BPH/LUTS should be routinely screened for PCa using serial PSA testing.[9]

The role of 5ARI in the treatment of low-risk cancers, as currently evaluated in some studies,[60] is not within the scope of this article. It just should be said that 5ARI in the treatment of PCa is currently not a valid treatment option and should only be offered in the context of approved clinical trials.

5-ALPHA-REDUCTASE INHIBITOR COMBINATION THERAPY
Combination with Alpha-Blockers

Alpha-adrenergic receptor antagonists (ie, ABs) are still the first-line option in men with moderate to severe BPH/LUTS suitable for drug therapy.[9] This might be well explained by the high clinical efficacy of ABs, their low adverse side effect profile, their quick onset of action, and their low costs.[24,61,62] Looking into real-life practice patterns, ABs are by far the most commonly prescribed drugs for BPH/LUTS.[63,64] Among the different ABs available, there seem to be no meaningful clinical differences.[65] Combining ABs with 5ARIs not only holds the prospect to be more effective in terms of clinical BPH/LUTS improvement but also combines the quick onset of action of ABs with the long-term beneficial effects of reduced BPH progression of 5ARIs.

The first clinical studies combining 5ARIs with ABs in BPH/LUTS subjects were performed in Japan during the 1990s.[66,67] Since then, 6 larger randomized controlled trials assessing this combination have been performed: the Veterans Affairs Cooperative (VA-COOP) study[20]; the Alfuzosin, Finasteride, and combination in the treatment of BPH (ALFIN) study[68]; the Prospective European Doxazosin and Combination Therapy (PREDICT) study[22]; the Medical Therapy of Prostatic Symptoms (MTOPS) study[69]; CombAT[70]; and, just recently, the Comparative efficacy of Dutasteride plus Tamsulosin (CONDUCT) study.[71] Additionally, countless post hoc subgroup analyses to these trials have been published.

VA-COOP, ALFIN, and PREDICT could not demonstrate any advantage of 5ARI/AB combination over AB monotherapy in regard to IPSS or AUA-SS reduction, and Q_{max} increase; and no advantage over 5ARI monotherapy in regard to prostate size reduction.[72] VA-COOP, ALFIN, and PREDICT had study durations of less than 1 year (**Table 1**). MTOPS and CombAT, which lasted 4 to 6 years, showed significant advantages of 5ARI/AB combination over either monotherapy.[72] Apart from differences in the study designs, such as different primary end points, the different outcomes between short-term and long-term trials still suggest that the beneficial effects of 5ARI/AB combination do not occur before 1 year.[72]

In MTOPS, combination therapy changed AUA-SS by −7.4 compared with −6.6 for doxazosin (AB) or −5.6 for FIN alone.[69] In CombAT, IPSS was reduced by −6.3 in the combination group compared with −3.8 in the tamsulosin (TAM; AB), and −5.3 in the DUT group.[70] Different outcomes between MTOPS and CombAT are most likely explained by different study inclusion criteria. Whereas MTOPS included all subjects suffering from LUTS without any prostate size limitation (average prostate size at baseline 36 ± 20 mL), CombAT only included men with prostate sizes greater than 30 mL (average prostate size at baseline 55 ± 23 mL).[72] Different inclusion criteria might also explain different outcomes in Q_{max} between MTOPS and CombAT. Both studies showed, however, clear superiority of combination over either monotherapy in regard to Q_{max} improvement (see **Table 1**). In MTOPS, clinical progression was defined as an AUA-SS increase 4 or greater, AUR, renal insufficiency, recurrent urinary tract infections, or unacceptable incontinence episodes.[69] Within 4 years, clinical progression was experienced by 5% of subjects receiving combination therapy, by 10% receiving any monotherapy, and by 17% of PBO subjects.[69]

Post hoc analyses revealed that the bigger the prostate size was at study entry the more pronounced are the clinical effects of 5ARI/AB combination therapy.[73] In MTOPS, the overall NNT to prevent 1 subject from surgery was 25.9 for combination therapy and it dropped to 15.9 in those subjects who had a prostate size greater than 40 mL at baseline.[69] In CombAT, the relative risk reduction to develop AUR or BPH-related surgery with combination (compared with ABs alone) was 69.3% for subjects with a prostate size 42 to 57.8 mL and 72.6% for subjects with a prostate size greater than 57.8 mL.[73] However, not only was combination therapy clinically more effective in subjects with enlarged prostates, the time at which the superiority of combination over monotherapy became apparent was sooner in men with larger prostates.[72] In subjects with a prostate less than 42 mL, superiority of combination over AB monotherapy in regard to IPSS reduction became apparent at month 21, at month 6 in subjects with a prostate 42 to 58 mL, and at 3 months in subjects with a prostate greater than 58 mL.[27]

CONDUCT was the first trial to assess a single-capsule formulation of TAM/DUT (Duodart). The study included 742 men with moderate (not severe) LUTS (IPSS 8–19) and a prostate 30 mL or greater. Men were randomized to receive either TAM/DUT or watchful waiting (WW).[71] However, subjects in the WW group were switched to TAM monotherapy if IPSS increased or stayed the same on follow-up visits. Over 2 years of study duration, 61% of the WW group had to be switched to TAM, meaning that at study end comparisons were made between TAM/DUT and a composite group of WW and TAM (WW/TAM).[71] IPSS was −5.4 for TAM/DUT versus −3.6 for WW/TAM. The significant difference between TAM/DUT and WW/TAM started at month 1. Data on prostate size or Q_{max} were not reported.[71] Relative risk reduction for clinical progression was −43% for TAM/DUT versus WW/TAM. Side effects were higher for TAM/DUT than for WW/TAM, and similar to those reported in other studies.[71] The data indicate that in men with moderate LUTS and a prostate 30 mL or greater, TAM/DUT is more effective than WW or TAM.

Drug-related AEs and side effects occur significantly more often in the combination than in monotherapy groups (**Table 2**). However, the antiandrogenic AEs of 5ARIs and the known AEs of ABs, such as hypotension, dizziness, and rhinitis, are they are cumulative and not potentiated cumulative and do not seem to potentiate synergistically.[72] In CombAT, serious AEs occurred in less than 1% in each treatment arm and, after 4 years, only 6% of subjects in the combination group and 4% in the monotherapy groups had stopped taking medication due to

Table 1
Selected clinical outcomes of 5-alpha reductase inhibitor alpha-adrenergic antagonist combination therapy

Trial	Subjects	Duration (mo)	5-ARI	AB	IPSS or AUA-SS				Q_{max} (mL/s)				Prostate Size (mL or %)			
					5-ARI	AB	PBO	COM	5-ARI	AB	PBO	COM	5-ARI	AB	PBO	COM
VA-COOP	1229	12	FIN 5 mg	Terazosin 10 mg	−3.2	−6.1	−2.6	−6.2	+1.6	+2.7	+1.4	+3.2	−6.1	+0.5	+0.5	−7.0
ALFIN	1051	6	FIN 5 mg	Alfuzosin 2 × 5 mg	−5.2	−6.3	—	−6.1	+1.6	+1.8	—	+2.3	−4.3	−0.2	—	−4.9
PREDICT	1095	12	FIN 5 mg	Doxazosin 4–8 mg	−6.6	−8.3	−5.7	−8.5	+1.8	+3.6	+1.4	+3.8	—	—	—	—
MTOPS	3047	54–72	FIN 5 mg	Doxazosin 4–8 mg	−5.6	−6.6	−4.9	−7.4	+2.2	+2.5	+1.4	+3.7	−19%	+24%	+24%	−19%
CombAT	3822	24–48	DUT 0.5 mg	Tamsulosin 0.4 mg	−5.3	−3.8	—	−6.3	+2.0	+0.7	—	+2.4	−28%	+4.6%	—	−27%
CONDUCT	742	24	DUT 0.5 mg	Tamsulosin 0.4 mg	—	−3.6[a]	—	−5.4	—	—	—	—	—	—	—	—

— Means not reported or not assessed.

Abbreviation: COM, combination.

[a] A combined group of watchful waiting and tamsulosin monotherapy in CONDUCT.

Table 2
Selected side effects of 5-alpha reductase inhibitor alpha-adrenergic antagonist combination therapy

Trial	Dizziness and Hypotension				Impotence				Drug-Related AEs Total				Discontinuation Rates Due to Drug-Related AEs			
	5-ARI	AB	PBO	COM	5-ARI	AB	PBO	COM	5-ARI	AB	PLC	COM	5-ARI	AB	PBO	COM
VA-COOP	8%	26%	7%	21%	9%	6%	5%	9%	—	—	—	—	6.1%	7%	1.9%	9.4%
ALFIN	1.2%	1.7%	—	2.3%	6.7%	2.2%	—	7.4%	26%	27%	—	26%	5.9%	7.8%	—	8.1%
PREDICT	8%	15.6%	7.4%	13.6%	4.9%	5.8%	10.5%	3.3%	—	—	—	—	13.6%	11.6%	11.9%	12.6%
MTOPS	2.3%[b]	4.4%[b]	2.2%[b]	5.3%[b]	4.5%[b]	3.5%[b]	3.3%[b]	5.1%[b]	24%	27%	—	18%	—	—	—	—
CombAT	<1%	2%	—	2%	7%	5%	—	9%	21%	19%	—	28%	4%	4%	—	6%
CONDUCT	—	2%[a]	—	2%	—	0%[a]	—	8%	—	10%[a]	—	24%	—	5%[a]	—	7%

— Means not reported or not assessed.
Abbreviation: COM, combination.
[a] A combined group of watchful waiting and TAM monotherapy in CONDUCT.
[b] Rate per 100 person-years of follow-up.

AEs.[70] As a consequence, AEs are not considered a relevant criterion against combination therapy.[72]

Special attention, however, should be given to the sexual AEs of combination therapy. Potential sexual AEs of ABs, such as EjD, can sum up to the known antiandrogenic sexual AEs of 5ARIs and, therefore, even worsen the sexual satisfaction of patients.[72] According to a recent meta-analysis, the risk of EjD seems to be a threefold increase compared with AB or 5ARI monotherapy.[74] In addition, there have been reports that sexual dysfunction related to 5ARI intake might persist even when the 5ARI is stopped; however, these reports still to be confirmed.[75] Regardless of comorbidities and age, the risk for sexual dysfunction is clearly increased in BPH/LUTS patients with an odds ratio ranging from 1.39 to 2.67.[76] Therefore, the potential sexual AEs of combination therapy should particularly be openly discussed with a patient before starting therapy.

In summary, patients with enlarged prostates (>30–40 mL) and intended long-term treatment (>1 year) benefit from 5ARI/AB combination therapy if potential sexual AEs or intolerance towards ABs do not disqualify them from treatment.

Combination with Phosphodiesterase Type 5 Inhibitors

Phosphodiesterase type 5 inhibitors (PDE5Is), namely tadalafil (TAD; Cialis), which is the only PDE5I approved by FDA and the European Medicines Agency (EMA) for the treatment of BPH/LUTS, might be a real game changer. TAD was reported to be equally effective as ABs in the reduction of BPH/LUTS[77] and is believed to be a future alternative to AB treatment.[9] In addition, PDE5Is significantly increase erectile function.[78] Particularly because ED is a well-known side effect of 5ARI treatment, the combination of 5ARI with PDE5I seems appealing.

So far, only 1 clinical trial has reported on 5ARI/PDE5I combination. In this trial, 695 subjects aged 45 years or older, with an IPSS 13 or greater and a prostate volume 30 mL or greater received either PBO/FIN 5 mg or TAD 5 mg/FIN 5 mg combination over a 26-week period.[79] At study end, IPSS changed −4.5 for PBO/FIN and −5.5 for TAD/FIN.[79] International Index of Erectile Function, assessing erectile function, was ±0 with PBO/FIN, and +12 with TAD/FIN.[79] Regarding safety and tolerability, the TAD/FIN combination seems to be safe. There was 31% in the TAD/FIN and 27% in the PBO/FIN group that reported at least 1 treatment emergent AE, mostly mild to moderate in severity.[79]

Interestingly, discontinuation rates due to AEs were numerically higher with PBO/FIN than with TAD/FIN (2.3 vs 1.4%), even though this difference did not reach statistical significance. Subgroup analysis revealed that the beneficial effects of 5ARI/PDE5I combination on erectile function occurred regardless of whether or not subjects were suffering from ED at study initiation.[80]

In summary, initial data on 5ARI/PDE5I combination therapy seem very promising. However, this should be confirmed in larger and longer clinical trials before any recommendation is given.

SUMMARY

In men with BPH/LUTS, 5ARIs reduce prostate sizes up to 25%, increase Q_{max} approximately 1 to 3 mL/s, and decrease AUA or IP symptom scores approximately 2 to 5 points. However, only patients with an enlarged prostate (>30–40 mL) benefit significantly from 5ARI intake. The bigger the prostate is at study initiation, the faster the clinical effects of 5ARIs become apparent. Overall, it is reported that 5ARIs should be taken at least a year for the effects to become significant. FIN and DUT seem to be equally effective with no meaningful clinical differences and no relevant differences in regard to side effects. Clinically relevant side effects of 5ARIs mainly affect sex life with ED, EjDs, and loss of libido. Potential sexual side effects of 5ARI should be openly discussed with patients before therapy commencement.

In healthy men, within 7 years, 5ARIs were shown to decrease prostate cancer incidence by 25%. However, there was also a significant increase of high-grade cancers with 5ARIs, leading to the conclusion that there is no acceptable risk-benefit ratio for 5ARIs in PCa prevention. Even though large observational studies showed no higher occurrence of PCa or mortality rate with 5ARIs, BPH patients undergoing 5ARI treatment should be routinely screened for PCa. Because 5ARIs affect PSA levels, PSA values should be doubled if used for PCa screening.

Combination of 5ARI with an AB is faster in its clinical onset of action, and more effective than any monotherapy in regard to symptom score reduction, Q_{max} improvement, and reduction of clinical progression. With 5ARI/AB combination the relative risk reduction for clinical progression or the need for prostate surgery reaches 66%. 5ARI/AB combination therapy is recommended in patients with a prostate greater than 30 to 40 mL, and an intended drug therapy greater than 1 year, if they are otherwise suitable for AB therapy. Side effects, particularly sexual side effects, occur more frequently with 5ARI/AB combination therapy than with either monotherapy. The initial data on 5ARI/PDE5I combination are very promising but more and longer trials are needed to better evaluate this therapeutic option.

REFERENCES

1. Azzouni F, Godoy A, Li Y, et al. The 5 alpha-reductase isozyme family: a review of basic biology and their role in human diseases. Adv Urol 2012; 2012:530121.
2. Wilson JD. Role of dihydrotestosterone in androgen action. Prostate Suppl 1996;6:88–92.
3. Imperato-McGinley J, Peterson RE, Gautier T, et al. Androgens and the evolution of male-gender identity among male pseudohermaphrodites with 5alpha-reductase deficiency. N Engl J Med 1979;300(22): 1233–7.
4. Huggins C, Steven R. The effect of castration on benign hypertrophy of the prostate in man. J Urol 1940;43:705–14.
5. Wilson JD. Recent studies on the mechanism of action of testosterone. N Engl J Med 1972;287(25): 1284–91.
6. Wilson JD. The pathogenesis of benign prostatic hyperplasia. Am J Med 1980;68(5):745–56.
7. Marks LS. 5alpha-reductase: history and clinical importance. Rev Urol 2004;6(Suppl 9):S11–21.
8. McVary KT, Roehrborn CG, Avins AL, et al. Update on AUA guideline on the management of benign prostatic hyperplasia. J Urol 2011;185(5):1793–803.
9. Oelke M, Bachmann A, Descazeaud A, et al. EAU guidelines on the treatment and follow-up of non-neurogenic male lower urinary tract symptoms including benign prostatic obstruction. Eur Urol 2013;64(1):118–40.
10. Stoner E. The clinical development of a 5 alpha-reductase inhibitor, finasteride. J Steroid Biochem Mol Biol 1990;37(3):375–8.
11. Rittmaster RS, Stoner E, Thompson DL, et al. Effect of MK-906, a specific 5 alpha-reductase inhibitor, on serum androgens and androgen conjugates in normal men. J Androl 1989;10(4):259–62.
12. Vermeulen A, Giagulli VA, De Schepper P, et al. Hormonal effects of an orally active 4-azasteroid inhibitor of 5 alpha-reductase in humans. Prostate 1989;14(1):45–53.
13. McConnell JD, Wilson JD, George FW, et al. Finasteride, an inhibitor of 5 alpha-reductase, suppresses prostatic dihydrotestosterone in men with benign prostatic hyperplasia. J Clin Endocrinol Metab 1992;74(3):505–8.
14. Gormley GJ, Stoner E, Bruskewitz RC, et al. The effect of finasteride in men with benign prostatic hyperplasia. The Finasteride Study Group. N Engl J Med 1992;327(17):1185–91.
15. Hudson PB, Boake R, Trachtenberg J, et al. Efficacy of finasteride is maintained in patients with benign prostatic hyperplasia treated for 5 years. The North American Finasteride Study Group. Urology 1999; 53(4):690–5.
16. McConnell JD, Bruskewitz R, Walsh P, et al. The effect of finasteride on the risk of acute urinary retention and the need for surgical treatment among men with benign prostatic hyperplasia. Finasteride Long-Term Efficacy and Safety Study Group. N Engl J Med 1998;338(9):557–63.
17. Roehrborn CG, Bruskewitz R, Nickel JC, et al. Sustained decrease in incidence of acute urinary retention and surgery with finasteride for 6 years in men with benign prostatic hyperplasia. J Urol 2004; 171(3):1194–8.
18. Andersen JT, Ekman P, Wolf H, et al. Can finasteride reverse the progress of benign prostatic hyperplasia? A two-year placebo-controlled study. The Scandinavian BPH Study Group. Urology 1995;46(5): 631–7.
19. Nickel JC, Fradet Y, Boake RC, et al. Efficacy and safety of finasteride therapy for benign prostatic hyperplasia: results of a 2-year randomized controlled trial (the PROSPECT study). PROscar Safety Plus Efficacy Canadian Two year Study. CMAJ 1996; 155(9):1251–9.
20. Lepor H, Williford WO, Barry MJ, et al. The efficacy of terazosin, finasteride, or both in benign prostatic hyperplasia. Veterans Affairs Cooperative Studies Benign Prostatic Hyperplasia Study Group. N Engl J Med 1996;335(8):533–9.
21. Marberger MJ. Long-term effects of finasteride in patients with benign prostatic hyperplasia: a double-blind, placebo-controlled, multicenter study. PROWESS Study Group. Urology 1998; 51(5):677–86.
22. Kirby RS, Roehrborn C, Boyle P, et al. Efficacy and tolerability of doxazosin and finasteride, alone or in combination, in treatment of symptomatic benign prostatic hyperplasia: the Prospective European Doxazosin and Combination Therapy (PREDICT) trial. Urology 2003;61(1):119–26.
23. Boyle P, Gould AL, Roehrborn CG. Prostate volume predicts outcome of treatment of benign prostatic hyperplasia with finasteride: meta-analysis of randomized clinical trials. Urology 1996;48(3):398–405.
24. Tacklind J, Fink HA, Macdonald R, et al. Finasteride for benign prostatic hyperplasia. Cochrane Database Syst Rev 2010;(10):CD006015.
25. Roehrborn CG, Boyle P, Nickel JC, et al. Efficacy and safety of a dual inhibitor of 5-alpha-reductase types 1 and 2 (dutasteride) in men with benign prostatic hyperplasia. Urology 2002;60(3):434–41.

26. Roehrborn CG, Marks LS, Fenter T, et al. Efficacy and safety of dutasteride in the four-year treatment of men with benign prostatic hyperplasia. Urology 2004;63(4):709–15.

27. Roehrborn CG, Siami P, Barkin J, et al. The influence of baseline parameters on changes in international prostate symptom score with dutasteride, tamsulosin, and combination therapy among men with symptomatic benign prostatic hyperplasia and an enlarged prostate: 2-year data from the CombAT study. Eur Urol 2009;55(2):461–71.

28. Toren P, Margel D, Kulkarni G, et al. Effect of dutasteride on clinical progression of benign prostatic hyperplasia in asymptomatic men with enlarged prostate: a post hoc analysis of the REDUCE study. BMJ 2013;346:f2109.

29. Gittelman M, Ramsdell J, Young J, et al. Dutasteride improves objective and subjective disease measures in men with benign prostatic hyperplasia and modest or severe prostate enlargement. J Urol 2006;176(3):1045–50 [discussion: 1050].

30. Nickel JC, Gilling P, Tammela TL, et al. Comparison of dutasteride and finasteride for treating benign prostatic hyperplasia: the Enlarged Prostate International Comparator Study (EPICS). BJU Int 2011; 108(3):388–94.

31. Traish AM, Hassani J, Guay AT, et al. Adverse side effects of 5alpha-reductase inhibitors therapy: persistent diminished libido and erectile dysfunction and depression in a subset of patients. J Sex Med 2011;8(3):872–84.

32. Kaplan SA, Chung DE, Lee RK, et al. A 5-year retrospective analysis of 5alpha-reductase inhibitors in men with benign prostatic hyperplasia: finasteride has comparable urinary symptom efficacy and prostate volume reduction, but less sexual side effects and breast complications than dutasteride. Int J Clin Pract 2012;66(11):1052–5.

33. Wessells H, Roy J, Bannow J, et al. Incidence and severity of sexual adverse experiences in finasteride and placebo-treated men with benign prostatic hyperplasia. Urology 2003;61(3):579–84.

34. Schulman C, Pommerville P, Hofner K, et al. Long-term therapy with the dual 5alpha-reductase inhibitor dutasteride is well tolerated in men with symptomatic benign prostatic hyperplasia. BJU Int 2006;97(1):73–9 [discussion: 79–80].

35. Oelke M, Becher K, Castro-Diaz D, et al. Appropriateness of oral drugs for long-term treatment of lower urinary tract symptoms in older persons: results of a systematic literature review and international consensus validation process (LUTS-FORTA 2014). Age Ageing 2015;44(5):745–55.

36. Amory JK, Anawalt BD, Matsumoto AM, et al. The effect of 5alpha-reductase inhibition with dutasteride and finasteride on bone mineral density, serum lipoproteins, hemoglobin, prostate specific antigen and sexual function in healthy young men. J Urol 2008; 179(6):2333–8.

37. Lim SY, Laengvejkal P, Panikkath R, et al. The association of alpha-blockers and 5-alpha reductase inhibitors in benign prostatic hyperplasia with fractures. Am J Med Sci 2014;347(6):463–71.

38. Borst SE, Yarrow JF, Conover CF, et al. Musculoskeletal and prostate effects of combined testosterone and finasteride administration in older hypogonadal men: a randomized, controlled trial. Am J Physiol Endocrinol Metab 2014;306(4):E433–42.

39. Kacker R, Harisaran V, Given L, et al. Dutasteride in men receiving testosterone therapy: a randomised, double-blind study. Andrologia 2015;47(2):148–52.

40. Mella JM, Perret MC, Manzotti M, et al. Efficacy and safety of finasteride therapy for androgenetic alopecia: a systematic review. Arch Dermatol 2010; 146(10):1141–50.

41. Foley SJ, Soloman LZ, Wedderburn AW, et al. A prospective study of the natural history of hematuria associated with benign prostatic hyperplasia and the effect of finasteride. J Urol 2000;163(2):496–8.

42. Vasdev N, Kumar A, Veeratterapillay R, et al. Hematuria secondary to benign prostatic hyperplasia: retrospective analysis of 166 men identified in a single one stop hematuria clinic. Curr Urol 2013;6(3): 146–9.

43. Badawy AA, Abdelhafez AA, Abuzeid AM. Finasteride for treatment of refractory hemospermia: prospective placebo-controlled study. Int Urol Nephrol 2012;44(2):371–5.

44. Sandfeldt L, Bailey DM, Hahn RG. Blood loss during transurethral resection of the prostate after 3 months of treatment with finasteride. Urology 2001;58(6): 972–6.

45. Crea G, Sanfilippo G, Anastasi G, et al. Pre-surgical finasteride therapy in patients treated endoscopically for benign prostatic hyperplasia. Urol Int 2005;74(1):51–3.

46. Ozdal OL, Ozden C, Benli K, et al. Effect of short-term finasteride therapy on peroperative bleeding in patients who were candidates for transurethral resection of the prostate (TUR-P): a randomized controlled study. Prostate Cancer Prostatic Dis 2005;8(3):215–8.

47. Pastore AL, Mariani S, Barrese F, et al. Transurethral resection of prostate and the role of pharmacological treatment with dutasteride in decreasing surgical blood loss. J Endourol 2013;27(1):68–70.

48. Busetto GM, Giovannone R, Antonini G, et al. Short-term pretreatment with a dual 5alpha-reductase inhibitor before bipolar transurethral resection of the prostate (B-TURP): evaluation of prostate vascularity and decreased surgical blood loss in large prostates. BJU Int 2015;116(1):117–23.

49. Sato R, Sadaoka Y, Nishio K, et al. Effects of preoperative dutasteride treatment in holmium laser

enucleation of the prostate. Int J Urol 2015;22(4): 385–8.

50. Zhu YP, Dai B, Zhang HL, et al. Impact of preoperative 5alpha-reductase inhibitors on perioperative blood loss in patients with benign prostatic hyperplasia: a meta-analysis of randomized controlled trials. BMC Urol 2015;15:47.

51. Parsons JK, Schenk JM, Arnold KB, et al. Finasteride reduces the risk of incident clinical benign prostatic hyperplasia. Eur Urol 2012;62(2):234–41.

52. Oesterling JE, Roy J, Agha A, et al. Biologic variability of prostate-specific antigen and its usefulness as a marker for prostate cancer: effects of finasteride. The Finasteride PSA Study Group. Urology 1997;50(1):13–8.

53. Andriole GL, Guess HA, Epstein JI, et al. Treatment with finasteride preserves usefulness of prostate-specific antigen in the detection of prostate cancer: results of a randomized, double-blind, placebo-controlled clinical trial. PLESS Study Group. Proscar Long-term Efficacy and Safety Study. Urology 1998; 52(2):195–201 [discussion: 201–2].

54. Andriole GL, Marberger M, Roehrborn CG. Clinical usefulness of serum prostate specific antigen for the detection of prostate cancer is preserved in men receiving the dual 5alpha-reductase inhibitor dutasteride. J Urol 2006;175(5):1657–62.

55. Etzioni RD, Howlader N, Shaw PA, et al. Long-term effects of finasteride on prostate specific antigen levels: results from the prostate cancer prevention trial. J Urol 2005;174(3):877–81.

56. Thompson IM, Goodman PJ, Tangen CM, et al. The influence of finasteride on the development of prostate cancer. N Engl J Med 2003;349(3):215–24.

57. Andriole GL, Bostwick DG, Brawley OW, et al. Effect of dutasteride on the risk of prostate cancer. N Engl J Med 2010;362(13):1192–202.

58. Theoret MR, Ning YM, Zhang JJ, et al. The risks and benefits of 5alpha-reductase inhibitors for prostate-cancer prevention. N Engl J Med 2011; 365(2):97–9.

59. Preston MA, Wilson KM, Markt SC, et al. 5α-Reductase inhibitors and risk of high-grade or lethal prostate cancer. JAMA Intern Med 2014;174(8):1301–7.

60. Fleshner NE, Lucia MS, Egerdie B, et al. Dutasteride in localised prostate cancer management: the REDEEM randomised, double-blind, placebo-controlled trial. Lancet 2012;379(9821):1103–11.

61. Yuan JQ, Mao C, Wong SY, et al. Comparative effectiveness and safety of monodrug therapies for lower urinary tract symptoms associated with benign prostatic hyperplasia: a network meta-analysis. Medicine (Baltimore) 2015;94(27):e974.

62. DiSantostefano RL, Biddle AK, Lavelle JP. The long-term cost effectiveness of treatments for benign prostatic hyperplasia. Pharmacoeconomics 2006; 24(2):171–91.

63. Hutchison A, Farmer R, Verhamme K, et al. The efficacy of drugs for the treatment of LUTS/BPH, a study in 6 European countries. Eur Urol 2007; 51(1):207–15 [discussion: 215–6].

64. Hakimi Z, Johnson M, Nazir J, et al. Drug treatment patterns for the management of men with lower urinary tract symptoms associated with benign prostatic hyperplasia who have both storage and voiding symptoms: a study using the health improvement network UK primary care data. Curr Med Res Opin 2015;31(1):43–50.

65. Djavan B, Marberger M. A meta-analysis on the efficacy and tolerability of alpha1-adrenoceptor antagonists in patients with lower urinary tract symptoms suggestive of benign prostatic obstruction. Eur Urol 1999;36(1):1–13.

66. Okada H, Kawaida N, Ogawa T, et al. Tamsulosin and chlormadinone for the treatment of benign prostatic hyperplasia. The Kobe University YM617 Study Group. Scand J Urol Nephrol 1996;30(5):379–85.

67. Kuo HC. Comparative study of therapeutic effect of dibenyline, finasteride, and combination drugs for symptomatic benign prostatic hyperplasia. Urol Int 1998;60(2):85–91.

68. Debruyne FM, Jardin A, Colloi D, et al. Sustained-release alfuzosin, finasteride and the combination of both in the treatment of benign prostatic hyperplasia. European ALFIN Study Group. Eur Urol 1998; 34(3):169–75.

69. McConnell JD, Roehrborn CG, Bautista OM, et al. The long-term effect of doxazosin, finasteride, and combination therapy on the clinical progression of benign prostatic hyperplasia. N Engl J Med 2003; 349(25):2387–98.

70. Roehrborn CG, Siami P, Barkin J, et al. The effects of combination therapy with dutasteride and tamsulosin on clinical outcomes in men with symptomatic benign prostatic hyperplasia: 4-year results from the CombAT study. Eur Urol 2010;57(1):123–31.

71. Roehrborn CG, Oyarzabal Perez I, Roos EP, et al. Efficacy and safety of a fixed-dose combination of dutasteride and tamsulosin treatment (Duodart(®)) compared with watchful waiting with initiation of tamsulosin therapy if symptoms do not improve, both provided with lifestyle advice, in the management of treatment-naive men with moderately symptomatic benign prostatic hyperplasia: 2-year CONDUCT study results. BJU Int 2015;116(3):450–9.

72. Fullhase C, Chapple C, Cornu JN, et al. Systematic review of combination drug therapy for non-neurogenic male lower urinary tract symptoms. Eur Urol 2013;64(2):228–43.

73. Roehrborn CG, Barkin J, Siami P, et al. Clinical outcomes after combined therapy with dutasteride plus tamsulosin or either monotherapy in men with benign prostatic hyperplasia (BPH) by baseline characteristics: 4-year results from the randomized,

double-blind Combination of Avodart and Tamsulosin (CombAT) trial. BJU Int 2011;107(6):946–54.

74. Gacci M, Ficarra V, Sebastianelli A, et al. Impact of medical treatments for male lower urinary tract symptoms due to benign prostatic hyperplasia on ejaculatory function: a systematic review and meta-analysis. J Sex Med 2014; 11(6):1554–66.

75. Torre AL, Giupponi G, Duffy D, et al. Sexual dysfunction related to drugs: a critical review. Part V: alpha-Blocker and 5-ARI drugs. Pharmacopsychiatry 2016;49(1):3–13.

76. McVary K. Lower urinary tract symptoms and sexual dysfunction: epidemiology and pathophysiology. BJU Int 2006;97(Suppl 2):23–8 [discussion: 44–5].

77. Oelke M, Giuliano F, Mirone V, et al. Monotherapy with tadalafil or tamsulosin similarly improved lower urinary tract symptoms suggestive of benign prostatic hyperplasia in an international, randomised, parallel, placebo-controlled clinical trial. Eur Urol 2012;61(5):917–25.

78. Gacci M, Andersson KE, Chapple C, et al. Latest evidence on the use of phosphodiesterase type 5 inhibitors for the treatment of lower urinary tract symptoms secondary to benign prostatic hyperplasia. Eur Urol 2016. [Epub ahead of print].

79. Casabe A, Roehrborn CG, Da Pozzo LF, et al. Efficacy and safety of the coadministration of tadalafil once daily with finasteride for 6 months in men with lower urinary tract symptoms and prostatic enlargement secondary to benign prostatic hyperplasia. J Urol 2014;191(3):727–33.

80. Glina S, Roehrborn CG, Esen A, et al. Sexual function in men with lower urinary tract symptoms and prostatic enlargement secondary to benign prostatic hyperplasia: results of a 6-month, randomized, double-blind, placebo-controlled study of tadalafil coadministered with finasteride. J Sex Med 2015; 12(1):129–38.

Antimuscarinics, β-3 Agonists, and Phosphodiesterase Inhibitors in the Treatment of Male Lower Urinary Tract Symptoms
An Evolving Paradigm

Nadir I. Osman, PhD, MRCS[a], Reem Aldamanhori, MD, MBBS, SB-Urol[a,b],
Altaf Mangera, MBChB, MD, FRCS (Urol)[a],
Christopher R. Chapple, BSc, MD, FRCS (Urol), FEBU[a,*]

KEYWORDS

- Lower urinary tract symptoms • Storage LUTS • Phosphodiesterase inhibitors • Antimuscarinics
- β-3 Agonists

KEY POINTS

- Storage lower urinary tract symptoms (LUTS; including overactive bladder [OAB]) are most bothersome for patients and are likely to have an etiopathogenesis related to bladder function and abnormality affecting the bladder outlet.
- Several pharmacotherapies (antimuscarinics, β-3 agonist, and phosphodiesterase inhibitors) have emerged over the past decade, which show good efficacy and safety in the treatment of men with storage LUTS/OAB.
- The optimal place of these agents in the treatment algorithm will need to be decided by further studies assessing comparative efficacy and responder characteristics, with attention to the potential for combination therapy.

INTRODUCTION

Lower urinary tract symptoms (LUTS) occur frequently in older men[1] and are often bothersome with a negative impact on quality of life (QOL).[2] In most individuals, voiding and storage LUTS will coexist,[3] but storage LUTS are typically more bothersome.[4] Before the past decade, most therapeutic interventions were targeted at relieving voiding LUTS, through an effect on the prostate gland with the assumption that benign prostatic hyperplasia (BPH) was the main etiologic factor. In recent times, the influence of the bladder and in particular the afferent system on the development of storage LUTS has become widely accepted, which has changed the paradigm for the management of male LUTS away from a tradiational view of treating BPH, and the development

Conflicts of Interest: N.I. Osman has received speaker fees and an educational grant from Astellas. R. Aldamanhori has no conflicts of interest to disclose. A. Mangera has received speaker fees and an educational grant from Astellas. C.R. Chapple is a researcher and speaker for Astellas, Pfizer, Recordati, Lilly and Allergan.
[a] Department of Urology, Royal Hallamshire Hospital, Glossop Road, Sheffield S10 2JF, UK; [b] Department of Urology, University of Dammam, Bashar Ibn Burd Street, Khobar 31952, Kingdom of Saudi Arabia
* Corresponding author.
E-mail address: c.r.chapple@sheffield.ac.uk

Urol Clin N Am 43 (2016) 337–349
http://dx.doi.org/10.1016/j.ucl.2016.04.004
0094-0143/16/$ – see front matter © 2016 Elsevier Inc. All rights reserved.

urologic.theclinics.com

of new pharmacotherapeutic approaches has emerged.[5]

Overactive bladder (OAB) is a symptom complex that consists of an important and highly bothersome subset of storage LUTS and is defined as "urinary urgency with or without urgency incontinence usually accompanied by frequency and nocturia."[6] The sine qua non of OAB is urinary urgency, defined as "the sudden and compelling desire to void that is difficult to defer."[6] In men, OAB is often associated with detrusor overactivity, occurring in 69% and 90% of individuals with OAB without incontinence (OAB-dry) and OAB with incontinence (OAB-wet), respectively.[7]

Although for many years antimuscarinic agents were avoided in men due to the concern about causing urinary retention, there is now a strong evidence base to support the safety and efficacy of this class in treating male patients with storage LUTS/OAB. More recently, 2 new agents have been introduced into the therapeutic armamentarium in the treatment of male LUTS: the β-3 agonist and phosphodiesterase inhibitors. This article discusses the mechanism of action of these 3 agents in the context of the pathophysiology of LUTS/BPH in men before focusing on the evidence relating to their efficacy and safety.

ANTIMUSCARINICS
Mechanism of Action

Antimuscarinic agents act to some extent on the afferent (based on preclinical data) innervations, but probably principally on the parasympathetic (efferent) system. The chief functional receptor responsible for the motor activity of the detrusor muscle is the postjunctional muscarinic M_3 receptor.[8] Although the most numerous (75%) are the M_2 receptors, their function in the bladder along with that of M_4 and M_5 remains undefined.[9] The M_1 muscarinic receptors predominate in the central nervous system; M_1 and M_3 in salivary glands, M_2 and M_3 in the gastrointestinal tract, M_3 and M_5 in the eyes, and M_2 in the heart.[10]

M_3 receptor excitation leads to smooth muscle contraction via entry of extracellular calcium into the cell through L-type channels and activation of rho kinase.[11] Although there has been discussion about the potential importance of activity on M_2 receptors and sensory nerves and there is a body of literature to support this, these putative mechanisms of action still remain the subject of academic discussion.

In addition, neurotransmitters are released from the urothelium and suburothelium in response to distension and receptor activation.[12] Acetylcholine (Ach) has been shown to be released in greater amounts when the urothelium of bladder strips is intact, suggesting nonneuronal crosstalk between the urothelium and detrusor muscle.[13] It is also proposed that this nonneuronal Ach may enhance muscarinic receptor-mediated detrusor activity and may also be inhibited by antimuscarinic agents to different degrees.[14] Therefore, inhibition of smooth muscle "micromotion" may occur, a phenomenon that is postulated to occur because of leak of Ach from postganglionic parasympathetic nerve during the storage phase of micturition leading to activation of sensory afferent fibers and the sensation of urgency.[15] Recent work has also suggested that muscarinic activation also stimulates urothelial adenosine triphosphate release,[16] which may be of importance given that changes in purinergic signaling have been implicated in the aging bladder and are postulated to occur in bladder dysfunction.[17]

Current antimuscarinic agents approved by the regulatory authorities include oxybutynin, tolterodine, solifenacin, darifenacin, trospium, propiverine, and fesoterodine. The above antimuscarinic agents have different affinities for the different muscarinic receptors,[18] and darifenacin is the only agent with a high selectivity for the M_3 receptor over M_2.[19] Fesoterodine is an oral antimuscarinic drug that is metabolized rapidly and extensively to 5-hydroxymethyl tolterodine, the main active metabolite of tolterodine.[20] Tolterodine and its 5-hydroxymethyl metabolite (fesoterodine) do not discriminate between the receptor subtypes. Oxybutynin and solifenacin show fractional selectivity for M_3 receptors.

In animal models, greater bladder selectivity has been shown for tolterodine,[21] darifenacin,[22] and solifenacin[23] compared with oxybutynin. It should be noted that animal studies cannot be translated directly to the human situation, and this data should be interpreted with that in mind. Trospium chloride is a quaternary amine that is incompletely absorbed or metabolized, and the majority is excreted in the urine and therefore has a high bioavailability.[24] In addition to antimuscarinic activity, propiverine has been shown to antagonize Ca^{2+} channels, which may suppress smooth muscle contraction resistant to atropine.[25]

Clinical Efficacy

Two meta-analyses have reviewed anticholinergic medication use in patients with LUTS.[26,27] Some of the drugs are available as immediate release or once daily preparations, such as oxybutynin, propiverine, tolterodine, and trospium. In addition, oxybutynin is available as a transdermal patch and as a topical gel. Most of the trials in the meta-analyses had a placebo arm, and patient inclusion criteria were often diverse. The proportion of patients having received prior therapy was also variable. Median follow-up was 12 weeks.

The Chapple meta-analysis reported pooled differences, which showed a reduction of 0.5 to 1.3 micturition episodes per day and 0.4 to 1.1 incontinence episodes per day. Some trials reported changes in urodynamic parameters, such as the maximum cystometric capacity, which increased by 90 mL on average. In addition to this, QOL questionnaires, such as the Incontinence Impact Questionnaire, King's Health Questionnaire, and Urogenital Distress Inventory, were used to show significant benefits over placebo.

With very few trials comparing selective antimuscarinic agents against each other, a meta-analysis of these was not possible. Most patients in the randomized controlled trials (RCTs) were women, and men with a post void residual (PVR) urine volume of more than 200 mL were mostly excluded. This cutoff is rather arbitrary because there are no clear data to support that this is the clinically relevant threshold. In addition, men with voiding symptoms and poor flow were also excluded in most of the trials.

Given most patients in OAB trials are women, urologists have debated the utility of antimuscarinics in men; this is especially important given the potential risk of precipitating urinary retention. The TIMES (The tolterodine and tamsulosin in men with LUTS including OAB: evaluation and efficacy study) trial randomized men with both storage and voiding LUTS to tamsulosin or tolterodine monotherapy or a combination.[28] A PVR greater than 200 was an exclusion criterion. By 12 weeks, tolterodine monotherapy significantly reduced urgency urinary incontinence episodes versus placebo, but no other parameters were improved. By comparison, combination therapy led to significant reductions in OAB symptom outcomes, including bladder diary variables, International Prostate Symptom Score (IPSS) total, and storage subscores, including reduction in each of the individual storage symptom scores.

In another study, Kaplan and colleagues[29] were unable to demonstrate efficacy with tolterodine in men with storage symptoms. However, Herschorn and colleagues[30] have conducted a meta-analysis of fesoterodine 4 and 8 mg and found a reduction in frequency, urgency, and voided volumes. The risk of retention was not apparently increased in these. Solifenacin has also been shown to be efficacious in men with LUTS.[31]

Kaplan and colleagues[32] have systematically reviewed the evidence for antimuscarinics in men and reported a rate of urinary retention in less than 3% with nonsignificant changes in post void residue. A combination of antimuscarinic and α-antagonist was found to lead to greater symptomatic improvements than antimuscarinics alone, although antimuscarinics alone are efficacious and safe. The variable results with antimuscarinic agents alone probably boil down to patient selection and whether the patient has an element of bladder outlet obstruction contributing to their symptoms.

Combination therapy is considered a useful treatment option in men with both storage and voiding symptoms. Seven RCTs have shown the superiority of combination treatment over single-agent treatment and placebo. It is argued that the symptomatic differences are small but significant. Also, a trial powered to assess perception of treatment benefit showed a significant difference, suggesting this difference is still important to patients.[33]

Combination therapy has been investigated as sequential therapy, like in the ADAM (The tolterodine XL ADd-on to an Alpa-blocker in Men) and VICTOR (Vesicare in combination with tamsulosin in overactive bladder residual symptoms) studies, where the antimuscarinic was added later to tamsulosin or as a combination strategy from the outset, such as in the NEPTUNE (Study of Solifenacin Succinate and Tamsulosin Hydrochloride OCAS [oral controlled absorption system] in Males with Lower Urinary Tract Symptoms) study.[34–36] Sequential therapy is useful in men where the α-antagonist has not alleviated the patients' storage symptoms.

In the ADAM study, a significant advantage over placebo was found in total number of voids, day and nighttime frequency, Overactive bladder questionnaire (OAB-q) symptoms scores, and IPSS storage subscore.[34] In terms of total urgency episodes, there was a significant improvement in the add-on antimuscarinic group compared with placebo (-2.9 vs -1.8; $P = .0010$).

In the VICTOR study, a significant reduction in total number of urgency episodes for solifenacin/tamsulosin versus solifenacin/placebo was observed (-2.18 vs -1.10, $P<.001$), although there was no statistically significant difference between the groups in terms of total number of voids.[35] Approximately 1.5% of the tamsulosin/solifenacin group developed acute urinary retention (AUR) versus none in the tamsulosin/placebo group.

The NEPTUNE study was interesting because it included men with urodynamically proven bladder outlet obstruction with storage and voiding symptoms.[36] Men received solifenacin 6 or 9 mg with 0.4 mg tamsulosin. At 12 weeks, there was no significant difference in terms of Qmax, Pdet@Qmax, and bladder contractility index between the treatment groups and placebo.

A small randomized study including 107 men compared tolterodine, solifenacin, and darifenacin.[37] All 3 agents were effective in reducing total daily voids and IPSS. In terms of improvement in IPSS and urgency, tolterodine and solifenacin had an advantage over darifenacin. Overall, the PVR increased significantly (>50 mL) in the darifenacin group, while the rates of acute retention requiring catheterization and constipation were also higher, leading the investigators to conclude that darifenacin was not an optimal agent to use in men with LUTS/BPH. Further larger studies are needed to definitively establish whether there is differential efficacy across agents in this patient group.

Clinical Safety

The Chapple meta-analysis reported that trial withdrawal rate was only significant in patients taking oxybutynin immediate release at 15 mg/d and 7.5 to 10 mg/d over placebo and was not significant for any of the other drugs.[26] However, most RCTs are conducted over only a 12-week period, and the natural history of the OAB syndrome complex seems to fluctuate, probably because of its multifactorial nature. Therefore, discontinuation rates, which are obtained from after-market analysis, are actually up to 50%.[38,39]

In the mainstream trials included in the Chapple meta-analysis, dry mouth is the most commonly reported adverse event (AE) at 30% and 8% in treatment and placebo arms, respectively, followed by pruritus in 15% and 5%. In the meta-analysis, dry mouth rates were higher in active drug groups than the placebo groups. Other AEs included blurred vision, headache, constipation, erythema, fatigue, and urinary retention.

Meta-analysis of patients taking anticholinergic medications reported odds ratios of 1.36 for tolterodine, 1.93 for darifenacin, 2.07 for fesoterodine, 2.34 for oxybutynin, 2.93 for trospium, and 3.02 for solifenacin.[40] This meta-analysis suggests that the receptor selective agents may increase the risk of constipation over nonreceptor selective agents. The major limitation of this meta-analysis was the combination of nondirect comparison studies and the combination of data of different dosages and formulations.

Cognitive impairment is often not thoroughly assessed in many trials involving anticholinergic medications.[41] It is, however, considered to pose a significant risk in the elderly population and in those with conditions such as diabetes, Alzheimer disease, stroke, trauma, multiple sclerosis, and Parkinson disease because of increased permeability of the blood-brain barrier.[42] Therefore, this needs assessing in this at-risk population with longer-term studies.

Another consideration in men is the risk of precipitating urinary retention. The limitation of most studies is that they are short term (12 weeks) (Table 1), and also most studies excluded men with larger PVRs (usually >200 mL) who would be at higher risk due to a presumed reduction in the detrusor contractile function. Furthermore, in the

Table 1
Incidence of urinary retention in key studies of antimuscarinics in men with lower urinary tract symptoms

Study	Length (wk)	Patients (n)	Groups	Incidence of AUR Needing Catheterization (%)
Kaplan et al,[28] (TIMES)	12	879	Tolterodine	0
			Tamsulosin	0
			Tolterodine + Tamsulosin	<1
			placebo	<1
Chapple et al,[34] (ADAM)	12	652	Tolterodine ER + AB	<1
			Placebo + AB	<1
Kaplan et al,[35] (VICTOR)	12	398	Solifenacin + Tamsulosin	1.5
			Placebo + Tamsulosin	0
Macdiarmid et al,[33] 2008	12	420	Oxybutynin + Tamsulosin	0
			Placebo + Tamsulosin	0
Kaplan et al[36]	12	222	Solifenaciin + Tamsulosin	<1
			Placebo + Tamsulosin	0
Abrams et al[43]	12	221	Tolterodine	0
			Placebo	1.2

studies that measured prostate size, volumes were generally low. As such, antimuscarinics are generally not recommended in men with PVR greater than 200 mL, in men who have low peak flow rates, or in men who have larger prostates or a previous history of AUR.

In a population-based study, the relative risk of urinary retention was increased to 8.3 in the first 30 days after commencing antimuscarinic therapy and thereafter decreased to a relative risk of 2 with longer-term use.[44] These data need to be interpreted with a degree of caution, because the participant characteristics are unclear. In the 12-week RCTs with selected patients, the risk is reported at 1% to 2%. There remains a need for longer-term studies to better assess the risk of urinary retention and determine the safe upper limit in terms of baseline PVR.

Summary

Antimuscarinic agents have long been used to treat bladder storage symptoms in women. Their safety profile is well known among urologists. Similarly, their use in men is advocated by multiple RCTs. They are also beneficial in combination with an α-antagonist in men with mixed storage and voiding symptoms. In these men, they can be used as add-on therapy or as a combination with an α-antagonist from the outset. In men with urodynamically proven bladder outflow obstruction, they should only be used in combination.

The risk of urinary retention is low if men are selected appropriately as they are done for the RCTs. Specific exclusions should be PVR greater than 200 mL, Qmax 10 mL/s, large prostate, or a previous history of AUR.

β-3 AGONISTS
Mechanism of Action

Mirabegron is the first agent in a new therapeutic class introduced for the treatment of OAB that works by specific agonisms of the β-3 adrenoreceptor. Mirabegron is thought to enhance relaxation of the detrusor muscle and facilitate urine storage without affecting the detrusor contractile function during micturition. The detrusor relaxes mainly through the cyclic adenosine pathway, during which norepinephrine binds to the β-adrenoceptors. Within the detrusor muscle and the urothelial layer, 3 subtypes of β-adrenoceptors are present (β1, β2, and β3).[45] The vast majority are β3-adrenoceptors (more than 95%), which are thought to be the most important functionally.[46] The exact mechanism is not yet established but may include adenylyl cyclase activation with resulting increase in the intracellular cyclic adenosine phosphate as well as calcium channels.[47] It is currently hypothesized that a significant part of the efficacy is manifest on afferent pathways; hence, the apparent lack of voiding dysfunction in reported studies.

Clinical Efficacy

Several industry-sponsored studies conducted over the past 10 years have assessed the efficacy and safety of mirabegron in a total of more than 10,000 patients. The phase III program consisted of three 12-week double-blind placebo RCTs that took place in Europe, North America, and Australia.[48–50] Mirabegron was compared with a placebo or active comparator, tolterodine. The inclusion criteria consisted of adults (men and women older than the age of 18) with daytime frequency (≥8) and urgency with or without urgency incontinence (≥3 leakage episodes in a period of 3 days). The vast majority of patients studied were women (approximately 70%). The change in mean number of incontinence episodes and the mean number of micturitions in a 24-hour period were the primary end points. The mean number of urgency episodes per 24 hours and mean volume voided/micturition were the secondary endpoints.

Nitti and colleagues[51] presented results of a pooled analysis of efficacy data from the pivotal phase III studies. At 12 weeks, there was a significant reduction in the primary endpoint of mean incontinence episodes per 24 hours for mirabegron 50 mg and mirabegron 100 mg compared with placebo, −1.49, −1.50, and 1.10, respectively (P<.05). In terms of mean number of voids, reductions of −1.20, −1.75, and −1.74 were observed for placebo, Mirabegron 50 mg, and Mirabegron 100 mg, respectively (P<.05 for all comparisons). The mean number of micturitions per 24 hours was also significantly reduced for Mirabegron 50 mg and Mirabegron 100 mg compared with placebo, −0.55 and −0.54, respectively. For all the secondary endpoints of mean volume/micturition and mean number of urgency episodes (grade 3 or 4) per 24 hours, a significant reduction at 12 weeks for both doses of Mirabegron in comparison to placebo was noted. The higher dose of mirabegron did not add any discernible additional benefit over the lower dose.

Around half of the patients in the pooled analysis had had prior treatment with an antimuscarinic, which had been stopped due to either a lack of efficacy or a lack of tolerability. Mirbegron was efficacious in both those who had received prior antimuscarinics and those who had not.

Clinical Safety

The pooled analysis of safety data of the 3 pivotal phase III studies by Nitti and colleagues[51] showed the most common treatment-emergent adverse event (TEAE) to be hypertension and headache. These both occurred at a similar frequency to the both the placebo and the tolterodine groups. The development of dry mouth is one of the most bothersome TEAE with antimuscarinic therapy; the incidence of this problem with mirabegron (2%) was placebo level (2.1%), while with tolterodine it occurred 5 times as often (10.1%). Mirabegron was associated with approximate increases of 1 mm Hg or less in blood pressure and 1 bpm or greater in pulse rate as compared with placebo. Although these rates are acceptable, pharmacovigilance data will be essential in confirming safety in real life practice.

The 12-month study by Chapple and colleagues[52] demonstrated a similar incidence of TEAEs for mirabegron 50 mg, mirabegron 100 mg, and tolterodine ER 4 mg. Again dry mouth was more frequent in the tolterodine group (8.6%) in comparison to mirabegron (2.3%–2.8%). However, all the groups had a similar rate of subjects discontinuing the medication because of TEAEs, 6.4%, 5.9%, and 6.0% for mirabegron 50 mg, mirabegron 100 mg, and tolterodine ER 4 mg, respectively.

An important issue in men with LUTS is the risk of urinary retention; hence, in the phase III studies, PVR volume was included as a safety endpoint. In the pooled analysis, the overall occurrence of urinary retention was low, and lowest in mirabegron-treated patients (placebo 0.5%, mirabegron 25 mg 0%, mirabegron 50 mg 0.1%, mirabegron 100 mg 0%, tolterodine 0.5%). No clinically relevant changes in PVR, from baseline to last visit, occurred in any group. Similarly, in the 12-month study by Chapple and colleagues, the incidence of urinary retention was low across the groups, occurring in 1, 1, and 3 patients in the mirabegron 50 mg, mirabegron 100 mg, and tolterodine ER 4 mg groups. Nitti and colleagues[53] sought to further assess the effect of mirabegron on voiding parameters by assessing more than 200 men (>45 years) with LUTS and bladder outlet obstruction with urodynamic studies pretreatment and posttreatment with placebo or mirabegron. They found that mirabegron (50 or 100 mg) did not adversely affect maximal flow or detrusor pressure at maximal flow after 12 weeks of treatment.

Summary

Mirabegron was shown to be safe and effective in the treatment of patients with OAB. There is no evidence of a greater efficacy at the higher dose of 100 mg compared with 50 mg. Mirabegron was associated with levels of dry mouth similar to placebo, while the safety profile appears to be acceptable. Mirabegron is therefore a treatment option in patients with men with OAB, with or without a history of prior antimuscarinic use. Most patients studied in the phase III program are women, and so there is a need for further studies to better characterize the features of men who respond to treatment. In the future, it will be interesting to see whether the low rate of dry mouth translates to any significant difference in discontinuation rates compared with antimuscarinics in real clinical practice. However, there remains the important future need for adequate studies evaluating the use of this therapy in the male population affected by storage LUTS/BPH.

PHOSPHODIESTERASE INHIBITORS
Mechanism of Action

Both LUTS and erectile dysfunction (ED) are common conditions in aging men. The epidemiologic data, including national and multinational studies, suggest a strong correlation between ED and LUTS.[54] It has been proposed that the 2 problems may share a common pathophysiology. Postulated mechanisms include an alteration in the nitric oxide/cyclic guanosine monophosphate (NO/cGMP) signaling pathway.[55] NO produces smooth muscle relaxation effects by activating the soluble guanylate cyclase, subsequently increasing the tissue levels of cGMP, which in turn interact with various intracellular components that regulate activities of the contractile proteins. The role of the NO/cGMP pathway in relaxation of penile smooth muscle and erection is well understood. Numerous data suggest the presence of NO/cGMP-mediated regulatory functions of smooth muscle contractility in the bladder neck, urethra, and prostate.[56] NO-releasing nerves seem to be concentrated in the bladder outlet and cause cGMP-mediated relaxations.[57] Other possibilities include atherosclerosis in the pelvic vasculature, autonomic hyperactivity, and alterations in RhoA/Rho-kinase signaling.

Although it is well accepted that the enzyme phosphodiesterase-5 (PDE5) is expressed and is biologically active in the lower urinary tract (LUT), its functional role is still a matter of debate. Several mechanisms of action of PDE5-I in LUTS have been hypothesized.[58]

Induction of smooth muscle relaxation in the lower urinary tract
The NO/cGMP signaling pathway is thought to play a major role in the pathophysiology of LUTS/BPH. NO signaling occurs via stimulation of soluble guanylate cyclase producing cGMP. The level of cGMP in different LUT tissues can influence

the smooth muscle contractile ability and hence their capability to generate LUTS.[58] One way of changing cGMP levels is to selectively inhibit cGMP degradation. It is commonly agreed that PDE5-Is selectively inhibit the degradation of cyclic GMP. PDE5-Is increase the concentration and prolong the activity of intracellular cGMP; therefore, they reduce smooth muscle tone of the detrusor, prostate, and urethra.[59] Several in vitro studies have demonstrated that PDE5-Is can relax isolated prostate and bladder neck strips.[60,61]

Regulation of the proliferation and differentiation of lower urinary tract stroma

In the LUT (prostate, bladder, and urethra), PDE5 was virtually absent in the epithelial cells and expressed only in stromal cells.[62,63] The highest expression and biological activity of PDE5 was found in the bladder. However, a consistent PDE5 expression and activity were also found in prostatic urethra.[63] Tadalafil administration in rat models was associated with bladder antiproliferative and antifibrotic effects.[64,65] Several genes related to myofibroblast differentiation and fibrosis were downregulated in the bladder extracts or cells after tadalafil administration.

Affect afferent nerve activity

NO is suggested to also be involved in the micturition cycle, by inhibiting reflex pathways in the spinal cord and neurotransmission in the urethra, prostate, or bladder.[66] In spinal cord–injured patients, a single vardenafil administration achieved a significant decrease in maximum detrusor pressure and improvement in maximum cystometric capacity.[67] The NO/cGMP signaling pathway was proven to be involved in the regulation of the micturition reflex, with an action more predominant on the sensory rather than on the motor component with C-fiber afferent activation.[68]

Increasing lower urinary tract oxygenation

Immunohistochemical studies indicate that PDE5 is localized in the endothelial and smooth muscle cells of the LUT blood vessels.[63] It has also been proposed that PDE5-Is increase blood perfusion and oxygenation of the LUT, but the exact mechanism of action of PDE-Is remains to be determined.[69] Short-term administration of vardenafil and tadalafil increases bladder and prostate oxygenation.[70,71] Tadalafil was reported to improve impaired prostate and/or bladder perfusion.[65,72,73]

Regulating lower urinary tract symptoms–related inflammation

Metabolic syndrome and BPH/LUTS are often comorbid. Chronic inflammation is one of the acknowledged associations between these diseases. PDE5-Is hinder tumor necrosis factor-α (TNF-α)-induced inflammatory response in myofibroblasts.[74] PDE5-Is significantly reduce TNF-induced expression of inflammatory markers.[74]

Clinical Efficacy

Siaram and colleagues[75], in 2002, were the first to report the finding that PDE5 inhibition improved LUTS in men being treated for ED. Subsequently, evidence from RCTs of PDE5 inhibitor monotherapy in men with LUTS has shown significant reductions in IPSS scores versus placebo (**Table 2**).

Although RCTs on the efficacy of all 3 available oral PDE5-Is (sildenafil, tadalafil, and vardenafil) have been published during the last few years, only tadalafil (5 mg once daily) has been licensed for the treatment of male LUTS in Europe.[69] A meta-analysis reported that monotherapy with a PDE5-I achieved a significant improvement in the International Index of Erectile Function (IIEF) score (+5.5) and IPSS (−2.8), but no significant improvement in Qmax was found compared with placebo.[76]

The first systematic review on PDE5-Is for LUTS secondary to BPH published in the literature described a significant improvement of both urinary symptoms (IPSS decrease −2.8 to −6.3) and QOL change from baseline (−0.5 to −11.7) with a recognized effect on erectile function (IIEF +6.0 to +9.17).[77] With regard to tadalafil 5 mg, it was found that it significantly reduces IPSS by 22% to 37% (4.7–6.6 IPSS points).[78] Significant LUTS (IPSS) reduction has been documented with tadalafil as early as 1 week of treatment. Oelke and colleagues[78] also showed, for the first time, a significant increase in Qmax with tadalafil compared with placebo (+2.4 mL/s).

A further systematic review on all PDE5-Is demonstrated an improvement of ED (mean improvement of IIEF +4.0 to +6.9) with tadalafil 5 mg once daily, demonstrating a potential role for tadalafil in the treatment of men with coexistent BPH and ED.[79] A further meta-analysis demonstrated similar improvement of both urinary symptoms (IPSS −2.35 to −2.19) and erectile function (IIEF +4.93 to +4.66) in patients with BPH and those with coexistence of BPH and ED.[80]

Clinical Safety

In a recent review, the relative risk of AEs from tadalafil, vardenafil, and sildenafil was 2.27, 1.86, and 1.22, respectively. The overall incidence of TEAEs was 37.31% for PDE5-Is compared with 24.03% for placebo. Serious TEAEs were reported

Table 2
Summary of efficacy in key studies of phosphodiesterase-5-I in men with lower urinary tract symptoms

Study	No of Patients Completed (Active/Control)	Drug	Duration of F/U in wk	Outcome
Brock et al,[83] 2014	1496 (752/744)	T	12	The total treatment effect on total IPSS score improvement (2.25) was derived from a direct treatment effect of 1.57 and an indirect treatment effect of 0.67
McVary et al,[84] 2007	251 (125/126)	T	12	Significant improvement in • IPSS at 6 wk (−2.8 vs −1.2) • IPSS at 12 wk (−3.8 vs −1.7) Changes in uroflowmetry parameters were similar in the placebo and tadalafil groups
McVary et al,[85] 2007	323 (168/155)	S	12	Significant improvements in • IPSS (−6.32 vs −1.93) • BPH Impact Index (−2.0 vs −0.9) • Mean IPSS QOL score (−0.97 vs −0.29) There was no difference in urinary flow between the groups
Mulhall et al,[86] 2006	48	S	12	The mean improvement in the IPSS score was 4.6 points
Nickel et al,[87] 2015	1499 (752/747)	T	12	• Greater proportion of patients achieved a ≥3-point IPSS improvement (71.1% vs 56.0%) • ≥25% improvement in total IPSS randomization to endpoint (61.7% vs 45.5%)
Nishizawa et al,[88] 2015	1199 (601/598)	T	12	Significant improvement in total IPSS tadalafil vs placebo in • 4 wk (−3.69 vs −2.47) • 8 wk (−4.72 vs 3.43) • 12 wk (−5.32 vs −3.79)
Oelke et al,[89] 2015	1477 (742/735)	T	12	Clinically meaningful improvement (−3 IPSS points) from baseline to endpoint in significantly more patients with tadalafil (69.1%) vs placebo (54.8%)
Oelke et al,[90] 2014	1500 (752/748)	T	12	Tadalafil treatment resulted in reduction of −1 nocturia episodes in 47.5% of patients (vs 41.3% in placebo)
Porst et al,[91] 2009	491 (386/105)	T	12	• IPSS improvements were significantly greater for all tadalafil doses vs placebo • Changes in Qmax and PVR were small and not clinically meaningful
Porst et al,[92] 2011	300 (148/152)	T	12	Significant improvement in IPSS (−5.6 vs −3.6) Tadalafil did not significantly improve Qmax or reduce after-void residual volume
Porst et al,[93] 2013	1026 (505/521)	T	12	Significant improvement of total IPSS with tadalafil (−6.0) vs placebo (−3.6)

(continued on next page)

Study	No of Patients Completed (Active/Control)	Drug	Duration of F/U in wk	Outcome
Table 2 *(continued)*				
Porst et al,[94] 2013	1498 (752/746)	T	12	Improvements in IPSS and BPH-Impact Index in all patient subgroups
Roehrborn et al,[95] 2008	886 (701/185)	T	12	IPSS improved for: • 2.5 mg T (−3.9) • 5 mg T (−4.9) • 10 mg T (−5.2) • 20 mg T (−5.2) • vs placebo (−2.3) No statistically significant effect of treatment of peak flow at any tadalafil dose
Stief et al,[96] 2008	215 (105/110)	V	8	Significant improvement in • IPSS (−5.9 vs −3.6) Qmax and PVR urine volume did not change significantly with treatment

in 1.10%, 1.85%, and 1.05% of men treated with tadalafil, vardenafil, and sildenafil, respectively.[81]

The first meta-analysis looking at TEAEs due to PDE5-Is reported that flushing, headache, dyspepsia, and gastroesophageal reflux had the higher risk of occurrence. Comparably, flushing (4.37%), headache (4.23%), dyspepsia (3.69%), nasopharyngitis (2.27%), and dizziness (1.69%) were the most common treatment-related AEs in another meta-analysis.[82]

In a recent review on tadalafil once daily, a good safety profile with a relative risk of TEAEs from tadalafil comparable to those reported with vardenafil or sildenafil (2.27 vs 1.86 vs 1.22, respectively) was reported. Generally, the incidence of AEs reported was very similar to that stated with all PDE5-Is versus placebo (16.0% vs 6.0%).[79]

Summary

There is strong evidence for the improvement of LUTS/BPH with PDE5-Is. Because the prevalence of comorbid LUTS and ED in men with BPH is high, the treatment of both conditions with a single mode of therapy is of clinical interest. To date, only tadalafil 5 mg once daily has been officially licensed for the treatment of male LUTS, with or without ED. Therefore, only tadalafil should be used clinically for the treatment of male LUTS.[69]

SUMMARY

In 2016, there are several options available for the pharmacotherapeutic management of storage LUTS/OAB in men (**Fig. 1**). Antimuscarinics show

efficacy with an established evidence base for their safety. The main concerns are poor tolerability due to side effects such as dry mouth and the risk of retention in men with large residuals. A combination of antimuscarinic therapy with α-antagonist therapy has been reported to be effective. The introduction of the β -3 agonists may ultimately overcome both these limitations. However, more data are needed to directly compare these agents with antimuscarinics and to establish whether the preliminary data of studies of combination therapy of mirabegron and the antimuscarinic solifenacin represent a useful therapeutic approach for LUTS/BPH. It is important to assess what patient characteristics, if any, are predictive of a good response. PDE5-I has been shown to improve LUTS/BPH as well as erectile function, even though the exact

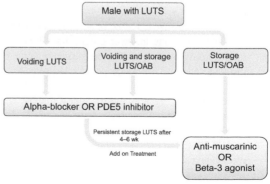

Fig. 1. Possible future male LUTS pharmacotherapy treatment algorithm.

mechanisms by which this is achieved is not established. The improvement in LUTS/BPH without a consistent concomitant improvement in Qmax suggests the mechanism of action is not simply the relief of bladder outlet obstruction (BOO). There are still many questions yet to be answered as to which agent should be used in which patient and at what stage before a definitive treatment algorithm can become established. There seems little doubt however that the traditional therapeutic approach with α-antagonists and 5-α reductase therapy has to be expanded to encompass these agents. Potentially, the future lies with varying combinations of therapy, building on the foundations of work with combined of α-antagonists and 5-α reductase therapy.

REFERENCES

1. Kupelian V, Wei JT, O'Leary MP, et al. Prevalence of lower urinary tract symptoms and effect on quality of life in a racially and ethnically diverse random sample: the Boston Area Community Health (BACH) Survey. Arch Intern Med 2006; 166(21):2381–7.

2. Coyne KS, Sexton CC, Kopp ZS, et al. The impact of overactive bladder on mental health, work productivity and health-related quality of life in the UK and Sweden: results from EpiLUTS. BJU Int 2011; 108(9):1459–71.

3. Sexton CC, Coyne KS, Kopp ZS, et al. The overlap of storage, voiding and postmicturition symptoms and implications for treatment seeking in the USA, UK and Sweden: EpiLUTS. BJU Int 2009; 103(Suppl 3):12–23.

4. Coyne KS, Wein AJ, Tubaro A, et al. The burden of lower urinary tract symptoms: evaluating the effect of LUTS on health-related quality of life, anxiety and depression: EpiLUTS. BJU Int 2009;103(Suppl 3):4–11.

5. Chapple CR, Roehrborn CG. A shifted paradigm for the further understanding, evaluation, and treatment of lower urinary tract symptoms in men: focus on the bladder. Eur Urol 2006;49(4):651–8.

6. Abrams P, Cardozo L, Fall M, et al. The standardisation of terminology in lower urinary tract function: report from the standardisation sub-committee of the International Continence Society. Urology 2003; 61(1):37–49.

7. Hashim H, Abrams P. Is the bladder a reliable witness for predicting detrusor overactivity? J Urol 2006;175(1):191–4 [discussion: 194–5].

8. Hegde SS, Eglen RM. Muscarinic receptor subtypes modulating smooth muscle contractility in the urinary bladder. Life Sci 1999;64(6–7):419–28.

9. Mansfield KJ, Liu L, Mitchelson FJ, et al. Muscarinic receptor subtypes in human bladder detrusor and mucosa, studied by radioligand binding and quantitative competitive RT-PCR: changes in ageing. Br J Pharmacol 2005;144(8):1089–99.

10. Abrams P, Andersson KE, Buccafusco JJ, et al. Muscarinic receptors: their distribution and function in body systems, and the implications for treating overactive bladder. Br J Pharmacol 2006;148(5): 565–78.

11. Schneider T, Fetscher C, Krege S, et al. Signal transduction underlying carbachol-induced contraction of human urinary bladder. J Pharmacol Exp Ther 2004;309(3):1148–53.

12. de Groat WC. The urothelium in overactive bladder: passive bystander or active participant? Urology 2004;64(6 Suppl 1):7–11.

13. Yoshida M, Inadome A, Maeda Y, et al. Non-neuronal cholinergic system in human bladder urothelium. Urology 2006;67(2):425–30.

14. Yoshida M, Masunaga K, Nagata T, et al. The forefront for novel therapeutic agents based on the pathophysiology of lower urinary tract dysfunction: pathophysiology and pharmacotherapy of overactive bladder. J Pharmacol Sci 2010;112(2):128–34.

15. Drake MJ, Mills IW, Gillespie JI. Model of peripheral autonomous modules and a myovesical plexus in normal and overactive bladder function. Lancet 2001;358(9279):401–3.

16. Sui G, Fry CH, Montgomery B, et al. Purinergic and muscarinic modulation of ATP release from the urothelium and its paracrine actions. Am J Physiol Renal Physiol 2014;306(3):F286–98.

17. Andersson KE. Muscarinic receptors and the aging bladder. In: Plas U, Pflüger U, Maier U, et al, editors. The ageing bladder. Vienna (Austria): Springer; 2004. p. 41–51.

18. Hegde SS. Muscarinic receptors in the bladder: from basic research to therapeutics. Br J Pharmacol 2006;147(Suppl 2):S80–7.

19. Fetscher C, Fleichman M, Schmidt M, et al. M(3) muscarinic receptors mediate contraction of human urinary bladder. Br J Pharmacol 2002;136(5):641–3.

20. Chapple C, Van Kerrebroeck P, Tubaro A, et al. Clinical efficacy, safety, and tolerability of once-daily fesoterodine in subjects with overactive bladder. Eur Urol 2007;52(4):1204–12.

21. Nilvebrant L, Andersson KE, Gillberg PG, et al. Tolterodine–a new bladder-selective antimuscarinic agent. Eur J Pharmacol 1997;327(2–3):195–207.

22. Gupta P, Anderson C, Carter ACJ, et al. In vivo bladder selectivity of darifenacin, a new M3 antimuscarinic agent, in the anesthetized dog. Eur Urol Suppl 2002;1(1):131–2.

23. Ikeda K, Kobayashi S, Suzuki M, et al. M(3) receptor antagonism by the novel antimuscarinic agent solifenacin in the urinary bladder and salivary gland. Naunyn Schmiedebergs Arch Pharmacol 2002;366(2): 97–103.

24. Doroshyenko O, Jetter A, Odenthal KP, et al. Clinical pharmacokinetics of trospium chloride. Clin Pharmacokinet 2005;44(7):701–20.

25. Zhu HL, Brain KL, Aishima M, et al. Actions of two main metabolites of propiverine (M-1 and M-2) on voltage-dependent L-type Ca2+ currents and Ca2+ transients in murine urinary bladder myocytes. J Pharmacol Exp Ther 2008;324(1):118–27.

26. Chapple CR, Khullar V, Gabriel Z, et al. The effects of antimuscarinic treatments in overactive bladder: an update of a systematic review and meta-analysis. Eur Urol 2008;54(3):543–62.

27. Novara G, Galfano A, Secco S, et al. A systematic review and meta-analysis of randomized controlled trials with antimuscarinic drugs for overactive bladder. Eur Urol 2008;54(4):740–63.

28. Kaplan SA, Roehrborn CG, Rovner ES, et al. Tolterodine and tamsulosin for treatment of men with lower urinary tract symptoms and overactive bladder: a randomized controlled trial. JAMA 2006;296(19):2319–28.

29. Kaplan SA, Roehrborn CG, Chancellor M, et al. Extended-release tolterodine with or without tamsulosin in men with lower urinary tract symptoms and overactive bladder: effects on urinary symptoms assessed by the International Prostate Symptom Score. BJU Int 2008;102(9):1133–9.

30. Herschorn S, Jones JS, Oelke M, et al. Efficacy and tolerability of fesoterodine in men with overactive bladder: a pooled analysis of 2 phase III studies. Urology 2010;75(5):1149–55.

31. Kaplan SA, Goldfischer ER, Steers WD, et al. Solifenacin treatment in men with overactive bladder: effects on symptoms and patient-reported outcomes. Aging Male 2010;13(2):100–7.

32. Kaplan SA, Roehrborn CG, Abrams P, et al. Antimuscarinics for treatment of storage lower urinary tract symptoms in men: a systematic review. Int J Clin Pract 2011;65(4):487–507.

33. MacDiarmid SA, Peters KM, Chen A, et al. Efficacy and safety of extended-release oxybutynin in combination with tamsulosin for treatment of lower urinary tract symptoms in men: randomized, double-blind, placebo-controlled study. Mayo Clin Proc 2008;83(9):1002–10.

34. Chapple C, Herschorn S, Abrams P, et al. Tolterodine treatment improves storage symptoms suggestive of overactive bladder in men treated with alpha-blockers. Eur Urol 2009;56(3):534–41.

35. Kaplan SA, McCammon K, Fincher R, et al. Safety and tolerability of solifenacin add-on therapy to alpha-blocker treated men with residual urgency and frequency. J Urol 2009;182(6):2825–30.

36. Kaplan SA, He W, Koltun WD, et al. Solifenacin plus tamsulosin combination treatment in men with lower urinary tract symptoms and bladder outlet obstruction: a randomized controlled trial. Eur Urol 2013;63(1):158–65.

37. Kaplan SA, Zoltan E, Te AE. Safety and efficacy of tolterodine, solifenacin, and darifenacin in men with lower urinary tract symptoms (LUTS) on alpha-blockers with persistent overactive bladder symptoms (OAB). J Urol 2008;179:701.

38. Lee YS, Choo MS, Lee JY, et al. Symptom change after discontinuation of successful antimuscarinic treatment in patients with overactive bladder symptoms: a randomised, multicentre trial. Int J Clin Pract 2011;65(9):997–1004.

39. Choo MS, Song C, Kim JH, et al. Changes in overactive bladder symptoms after discontinuation of successful 3-month treatment with an antimuscarinic agent: a prospective trial. J Urol 2005;174(1):201–4.

40. Meek PD, Evang SD, Tadrous M, et al. Overactive bladder drugs and constipation: a meta-analysis of randomized, placebo-controlled trials. Dig Dis Sci 2011;56(1):7–18.

41. Paquette A, Gou P, Tannenbaum C. Systematic review and meta-analysis: do clinical trials testing antimuscarinic agents for overactive bladder adequately measure central nervous system adverse events? J Am Geriatr Soc 2011;59(7):1332–9.

42. Kay GG, Ebinger U. Preserving cognitive function for patients with overactive bladder: evidence for a differential effect with darifenacin. Int J Clin Pract 2008;62(11):1792–800.

43. Abrams P, Kaplan S, De Koning Gans HJ, et al. Safety and tolerability of tolterodine for the treatment of overactive bladder in men with bladder outlet obstruction. J Urol 2006;175(3Pt1):999–1004.

44. Martín-Merino E, García-Rodríguez LA, Massó-González EL, et al. Do oral antimuscarinic drugs carry an increased risk of acute urinary retention? J Urol 2009;182(4):1442–8.

45. Andersson KE, Arner A. Urinary bladder contraction and relaxation: physiology and pathophysiology. Physiol Rev 2004;84(3):935–86.

46. Yamaguchi O. Beta3-adrenoceptors in human detrusor muscle. Urology 2002;59(5 Suppl 1):25–9.

47. Frazier EP, Peters SL, Braverman AS, et al. Signal transduction underlying the control of urinary bladder smooth muscle tone by muscarinic receptors and beta-adrenoceptors. Naunyn Schmiedebergs Arch Pharmacol 2008;377(4–6):449–62.

48. Khullar V, Amarenco G, Angulo JC, et al. Efficacy and tolerability of mirabegron, a beta(3)-adrenoceptor agonist, in patients with overactive bladder: results from a randomised European-Australian phase 3 trial. Eur Urol 2013;63(2):283–95.

49. Nitti VW, Auerbach S, Martin N, et al. Results of a randomized phase III trial of mirabegron in patients with overactive bladder. J Urol 2013;189(4):1388–95.

50. Herschorn S, Barkin J, Castro-Diaz D, et al. A phase III, randomized, double-blind, parallel-group, placebo-controlled, multicentre study to assess the efficacy and safety of the beta(3) adrenoceptor agonist, mirabegron, in patients with symptoms of overactive bladder. Urology 2013;82(2):313–20.

51. Nitti VW, Khullar V, van Kerrebroeck P, et al. Mirabegron for the treatment of overactive bladder: a pre-specified pooled efficacy analysis and pooled safety analysis of three randomised, double-blind, placebo-controlled, phase III studies. Int J Clin Pract 2013;67(7):619–32.

52. Chapple CR, Kaplan SA, Mitcheson D, et al. Randomized double-blind, active-controlled phase 3 study to assess 12-month safety and efficacy of mirabegron, a beta(3)-adrenoceptor agonist, in overactive bladder. Eur Urol 2013;63(2):296–305.

53. Nitti VW, Rosenberg S, Mitcheson DH, et al. Urodynamics and safety of the beta(3)-adrenoceptor agonist mirabegron in males with lower urinary tract symptoms and bladder outlet obstruction. J Urol 2013;190(4):1320–7.

54. Gacci M, Eardley I, Giuliano F, et al. Critical analysis of the relationship between sexual dysfunctions and lower urinary tract symptoms due to benign prostatic hyperplasia. Eur Urol 2011;60(4): 809–25.

55. McVary K. Lower urinary tract symptoms and sexual dysfunction: epidemiology and pathophysiology. BJU Int 2006;97(Suppl 2):23–8 [discussion: 44–5].

56. Köhler TS, McVary KT. The relationship between erectile dysfunction and lower urinary tract symptoms and the role of phosphodiesterase type 5 inhibitors. Eur Urol 2009;55(1):38–48.

57. Hedlund P. Nitric oxide/cGMP-mediated effects in the outflow region of the lower urinary tract–is there a basis for pharmacological targeting of cGMP? World J Urol 2005;23(6):362–7.

58. Gacci M, Andersson KE, Chapple C, et al. Latest evidence on the use of phosphodiesterase type 5 inhibitors for the treatment of lower urinary tract symptoms secondary to benign prostatic hyperplasia. Eur Urol 2016. [Epub ahead of print].

59. Uckert S, Oelke M, Stief CG, et al. Immunohistochemical distribution of cAMP- and cGMP-phosphodiesterase (PDE) isoenzymes in the human prostate. Eur Urol 2006;49(4):740–5.

60. Uckert S, Sormes M, Kedia G, et al. Effects of phosphodiesterase inhibitors on tension induced by norepinephrine and accumulation of cyclic nucleotides in isolated human prostatic tissue. Urology 2008;71(3):526–30.

61. Oger S, Behr-Roussel D, Gorny D, et al. Signalling pathways involved in sildenafil-induced relaxation of human bladder dome smooth muscle. Br J Pharmacol 2010;160(5):1135–43.

62. Filippi S, Morelli A, Sandner P, et al. Characterization and functional role of androgen-dependent PDE5 activity in the bladder. Endocrinology 2007;148(3): 1019–29.

63. Fibbi B, Morelli A, Vignozzi L, et al. Characterization of phosphodiesterase type 5 expression and functional activity in the human male lower urinary tract. J Sex Med 2010;7(1 Pt 1):59–69.

64. Maciejewski CC, Tredget EE, Metcalfe PD. Urodynamic improvements following oral medical therapy for partial bladder outlet obstruction in an animal model. Neurourol Urodyn 2015;34(3):286–91.

65. Kawai Y, Oka M, Yoshinaga R, et al. Effects of the phosphodiesterase 5 inhibitor Tadalafil on bladder function in a rat model of partial bladder outlet obstruction. Neurourol Urodyn 2016;35(4):444–9.

66. Andersson KE, Persson K. Nitric oxide synthase and the lower urinary tract: possible implications for physiology and pathophysiology. Scand J Urol Nephrol Suppl 1995;175:43–53.

67. Gacci M, Del Popolo G, Macchiarella A, et al. Vardenafil improves urodynamic parameters in men with spinal cord injury: results from a single dose, pilot study. J Urol 2007;178(5):2040–3 [discussion: 2044].

68. Caremel R, Oger-Roussel S, Behr-Roussel D, et al. Nitric oxide/cyclic guanosine monophosphate signalling mediates an inhibitory action on sensory pathways of the micturition reflex in the rat. Eur Urol 2010;58(4):616–25.

69. Oelke M, Bachmann A, Descazeaud A, et al. EAU guidelines on the treatment and follow-up of non-neurogenic male lower urinary tract symptoms including benign prostatic obstruction. Eur Urol 2013;64(1):118–40.

70. Morelli A, Filippi S, Comeglio P, et al. Acute vardenafil administration improves bladder oxygenation in spontaneously hypertensive rats. J Sex Med 2010; 7(1 Pt 1):107–20.

71. Morelli A, Filippi S, Sandner P, et al. Vardenafil modulates bladder contractility through cGMP-mediated inhibition of RhoA/Rho kinase signaling pathway in spontaneously hypertensive rats. J Sex Med 2009; 6(6):1594–608.

72. Yoshinaga R, Kawai Y, Oka M, et al. Effect of a single treatment with tadalafil on blood flow in lower urinary tract tissues in rat models of bladder overdistension/emptying and abdominal aorta clamping/release. Eur J Pharmacol 2015;754:92–7.

73. Vignozzi L, Filippi S, Comeglio P, et al. Tadalafil effect on metabolic syndrome-associated bladder alterations: an experimental study in a rabbit model. J Sex Med 2014;11(5):1159–72.

74. Vignozzi L, Gacci M, Cellai I, et al. PDE5 inhibitors blunt inflammation in human BPH: a potential mechanism of action for PDE5 inhibitors in LUTS. Prostate 2013;73(13):1391–402.

75. Sairam K, Kulinskaya E, McNicholas TA, et al. Sildenafil influences lower urinary tract symptoms. BJU Int 2002;90(9):836–9.

76. Gacci M, Corona G, Salvi M, et al. A systematic review and meta-analysis on the use of phosphodiesterase 5 inhibitors alone or in combination with α-blockers for lower urinary tract symptoms due to benign prostatic hyperplasia. Eur Urol 2012;61(5):994–1003.

77. Laydner HK, Oliveira P, Oliveira CR, et al. Phosphodiesterase 5 inhibitors for lower urinary tract symptoms secondary to benign prostatic hyperplasia: a systematic review. BJU Int 2011;107(7):1104–9.

78. Oelke M, Giuliano F, Mirone V, et al. Monotherapy with tadalafil or tamsulosin similarly improved lower urinary tract symptoms suggestive of benign prostatic hyperplasia in an international, randomised, parallel, placebo-controlled clinical trial. Eur Urol 2012;61(5):917–25.

79. Gacci M, Salvi M, Sebastianelli A, et al. The use of a single daily dose of tadalafil to treat signs and symptoms of benign prostatic hyperplasia and erectile dysfunction. Res Rep Urol 2013;5:99–111.

80. Dong Y, Hao L, Shi Z, et al. Efficacy and safety of tadalafil monotherapy for lower urinary tract symptoms secondary to benign prostatic hyperplasia: a meta-analysis. Urol Int 2013;91(1):10–8.

81. Liu L, Zheng S, Han P, et al. Phosphodiesterase-5 inhibitors for lower urinary tract symptoms secondary to benign prostatic hyperplasia: a systematic review and meta-analysis. Urology 2011;77(1):123–9.

82. Wang X, Li S, Meng Z, et al. Comparative effectiveness of oral drug therapies for lower urinary tract symptoms due to benign prostatic hyperplasia: a systematic review and network meta-analysis. PLoS One 2014;9(9):e107593.

83. Brock GB, McVary KT, Roehrborn CG, et al. Direct effects of tadalafil on lower urinary tract symptoms versus indirect effects mediated through erectile dysfunction symptom improvement: integrated data analyses from 4 placebo controlled clinical studies. J Urol 2014;191(2):405–11.

84. McVary KT, Roehrborn CG, Kaminetsky JC, et al. Tadalafil relieves lower urinary tract symptoms secondary to benign prostatic hyperplasia. J Urol 2007; 177(4):1401–7.

85. McVary KT, Monnig W, Camps JL Jr, et al. Sildenafil citrate improves erectile function and urinary symptoms in men with erectile dysfunction and lower urinary tract symptoms associated with benign prostatic hyperplasia: a randomized, double-blind trial. J Urol 2007;177(3):1071–7.

86. Mulhall JP, Guhring P, Parker M, et al. Assessment of the impact of sildenafil citrate on lower urinary tract symptoms in men with erectile dysfunction. J Sex Med 2006;3(4):662–7.

87. Nickel JC, Brock GB, Herschorn S, et al. Proportion of tadalafil-treated patients with clinically meaningful improvement in lower urinary tract symptoms associated with benign prostatic hyperplasia–integrated data from 1,499 study participants. BJU Int 2015; 115(5):815–21.

88. Nishizawa O, Yoshida M, Takeda M, et al. Tadalafil 5 mg once daily for the treatment of Asian men with lower urinary tract symptoms secondary to benign prostatic hyperplasia: analyses of data pooled from three randomized, double-blind, placebo-controlled studies. Int J Urol 2015;22(4):378–84.

89. Oelke M, Shinghal R, Sontag A, et al. Time to onset of clinically meaningful improvement with tadalafil 5 mg once daily for lower urinary tract symptoms secondary to benign prostatic hyperplasia: analysis of data pooled from 4 pivotal, double-blind, placebo controlled studies. J Urol 2015; 193(5):1581–9.

90. Oelke M, Weiss JP, Mamoulakis C, et al. Effects of tadalafil on nighttime voiding (nocturia) in men with lower urinary tract symptoms suggestive of benign prostatic hyperplasia: a post hoc analysis of pooled data from four randomized, placebo-controlled clinical studies. World J Urol 2014;32(5):1127–32.

91. Porst H, McVary KT, Montorsi F, et al. Effects of once-daily tadalafil on erectile function in men with erectile dysfunction and signs and symptoms of benign prostatic hyperplasia. Eur Urol 2009;56(4): 727–35.

92. Porst H, Kim ED, Casabé AR, et al. Efficacy and safety of tadalafil once daily in the treatment of men with lower urinary tract symptoms suggestive of benign prostatic hyperplasia: results of an international randomized, double-blind, placebo-controlled trial. Eur Urol 2011;60(5):1105–13.

93. Porst H, Roehrborn CG, Secrest RJ, et al. Effects of tadalafil on lower urinary tract symptoms secondary to benign prostatic hyperplasia and on erectile dysfunction in sexually active men with both conditions: analyses of pooled data from four randomized, placebo-controlled tadalafil clinical studies. J Sex Med 2013;10(8):2044–52.

94. Porst H, Oelke M, Goldfischer ER, et al. Efficacy and safety of tadalafil 5 mg once daily for lower urinary tract symptoms suggestive of benign prostatic hyperplasia: subgroup analyses of pooled data from 4 multinational, randomized, placebo-controlled clinical studies. Urology 2013;82(3):667–73.

95. Roehrborn CG, McVary KT, Elion-Mboussa A, et al. Tadalafil administered once daily for lower urinary tract symptoms secondary to benign prostatic hyperplasia: a dose finding study. J Urol 2008; 180(4):1228–34.

96. Stief CG, Porst H, Neuser D, et al. A randomised, placebo-controlled study to assess the efficacy of twice-daily vardenafil in the treatment of lower urinary tract symptoms secondary to benign prostatic hyperplasia. Eur Urol 2008;53(6):1236–44.

α-Blockers, 5-α-Reductase Inhibitors, Acetylcholine, β3 Agonists, and Phosphodiesterase-5s in Medical Management of Lower Urinary Tract Symptoms/Benign Prostatic Hyperplasia

How Much Do the Different Formulations Actually Matter in the Classes?

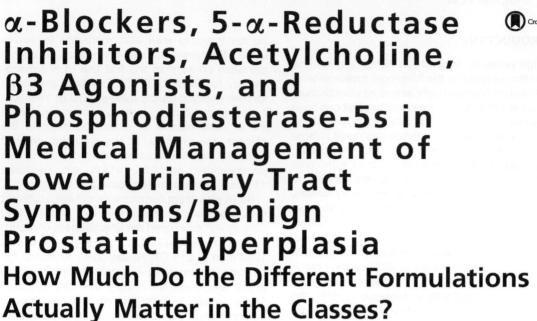

Bilal Chughtai, MD[a],*, Dominique Thomas, BS[a],
Steven Kaplan, MD[b]

KEYWORDS

- Benign prostatic hyperplasia • Lower urinary tract symptoms • Pharmacologic agents • α-Blockers
- 5-α-Reductase inhibitors (5ARIs) • β-3-Andrenoceptor agonists • Phosphodiesterase-5 inhibitors
- Anticholinergics

KEY POINTS

- The best pharmacologic agent and first line of treatment used to treat lower urinary tract symptoms (LUTS) secondary to benign prostatic hyperplasia (BPH) are α-blockers, which are rapid in alleviating symptoms.
- 5-α-Reductase inhibitors are the second line of defense for men presenting with large prostates and gradually work over months of monotherapy.
- Initial data support the use of phosphodiesterase-5 inhibitors (PDE5-Is) in treating BPH-LUTS, and PDE5-I is especially effective in cotreating concomitant erectile dysfunction.
- β-3-Andrenoceptor agonists and anticholinergics can be effective in treating overactive bladder and decreasing detrusor overactivity.
- Further studies are needed to evaluate head-to-head trials to assess the efficacy of the different class formulations.

[a] Department of Urology, Weill Cornell Medicine-New York, Presbyterian Hospital, 425 East 61st Street, 12th Floor, New York, New York 10065, USA; [b] Department of Urology, Mount Sinai Hospital, 625 Madison Avenue, 59th Street, 2nd Floor, New York, New York 10022, USA
* Corresponding author.
E-mail address: bic9008@med.cornell.edu

Urol Clin N Am 43 (2016) 351–356
http://dx.doi.org/10.1016/j.ucl.2016.04.013
0094-0143/16/$ – see front matter © 2016 Elsevier Inc. All rights reserved.

INTRODUCTION

Benign prostatic hyperplasia (BPH) is a medical condition defined as the histologic proliferation of epithelial and stromal cells as well as smooth muscle in the prostate.[1] It is a condition that can have bothersome effects on the patient's quality of life. The increase in prostatic tissue can result in large nodules in the transition zone of the prostate, which can lead to lower urinary tract symptoms (LUTS) involving a host of issues related to frequent urination, urgency, weak urinary stream, as well as other issues relating to voiding, storage, and postmicturition symptoms.[2,3] In the United States, about 50% of men older than 40 years of age will be diagnosed with this condition, and that percentage increases to 80% as men reach 80 years old.[1] Because of the degree of disease burden associated with a diagnosis of BPH, the incurred costs for appropriate medical management is well over $1.1 billion in the United States annually.[4] Over the last several decades, several treatment options have been introduced, such as surgical interventions, pharmacologic therapies, and the use of herbal remedies.

Following reports of randomized controlled trials (RCTs), the use of drug therapies has been associated with the standard of care for BPH-LUTS. These RCTs demonstrate the apparent effectiveness and safety when using the different drug classes and provide the physician with evidence of which class of drug is most effective depending on the presentation of symptoms. Currently, α-blockers, 5-α-reductase inhibitors (5ARIs), muscarinic receptor antagonists (MRAs), β3-agonists, and phosphodiesterase-5 inhibitors (PDE5-Is) have all been approved for treatment of BPH-LUTS and are widely recommended in clinical guidelines.[5] With a myriad of agents being approved for treatment a particular interest is their comparative effectiveness within their specific class. Many previous studies have compared the relative effectiveness between classes or in comparison to placebo groups. The objective of this study is to evaluate and compare the effectiveness of the different drug classes through head-to-head trials and provide a guide for physicians as to which treatments provide optimal results.

PHARMACOLOGIC TREATMENT OPTIONS

The following section compares various formulations for the treatment of LUTS secondary to BPH.

α-Blockers

The European Association of Urology current clinical guidelines state the use of α-blockers should be restricted to men with moderate to severe LUTS.[6] Furthermore, these pharmacologic agents are often considered the first line of pharmacotherapy for BPH-LUTS.[6,7] α-Blockers are known for their ability to rapidly relieve LUTS by interrupting the stimulation of α-adrenoceptors located on the smooth muscle in either the neck of the bladder, the prostate, or the prostatic urethra.[8] Currently, there are several different α-blockers commercially available, which are silodosin, alfuzosin, doxazosin, terazosin, and tamsulosin.

RCTs with direct comparisons between different α-blockers are minimal. However, Chapple and colleagues[9] compared the effectiveness of silodosin 8 mg, tamsulosin 0.4 mg, and a placebo among 1228 men in an RCT. Researchers evaluated the patient's International Prostate Symptom Score (IPSS) and maximum urinary flow rate (Qmax).[9] Those patients in both pharmacotherapy groups demonstrated statistical improvements in both IPSS scores and Qmax when compared with those in the placebo group.[9] Comparably, both silodosin and tamsulosin were equally effective in relieving the patient of LUTS; however, follow-up in those taking silodosin showed marked improvements in nocturia.[10] Furthermore, silodosin in comparison to other α-blockers is highly selective for α-1A andrenoceptor subtype over subtype 1B.[8,11] The high affinity of silodosin is thought to have a minimal prevalence for cardiovascular adverse events, but higher incidence of ejaculatory dysfunction.[8,9,11]

5-α-Reductase Inhibitors

In normal development, the growth of the prostate is regulated by the conversion of testosterone to dihydrotestosterone (DHT) by 5-α-reductase (5-AR) existing as type 1 and type 2.[12,13] Those with BPH tend to have an overabundance of DHT leading to BPH.[13] In order to combat this accumulation, the use of 5-AR inhibitors has been effective, and unlike α-blockers, has a direct effect on reducing the prostatic tissue.[13] The 2 main 5-AR inhibitors used for treating BPH/LUTS currently available are dutasteride and finasteride. The difference between the 2 is that dutasteride is capable of inhibiting both subtypes 1 and 2, whereas finasteride inhibits only subtype 2.[11] Nickel and colleagues[14] evaluated the effectiveness of dutasteride and finasteride in a head-to-had trial. This study, known as the Enlarged Prostate International Comparator Study (EPICS), was a multicenter randomized double-blind study of 1630 men older than the age of 50. Researchers found that both therapies were comparably effective in improving Qmax, reducing prostatic volume, and reducing other urinary symptoms in men with BPH when administered over a 12-month period.[14]

Kaplan and colleagues[15] retrospectively evaluated the safety, efficacy, and prostate volume (PV) over a 5-year period in BPH patients who were either treated with dutasteride or finasteride. Efficacy was evaluated using the following measures: peak urinary flow rate (Qmax), PV, postvoid residual urine volume (PVR), prostate-specific antigen (PSA), and IPSS.[15] From baseline to the 5-year mark, there were no significant differences in Qmax, PV, PVR, PSA, or IPSS for those in the finasteride group compared with those taking dutasteride.[15] Furthermore, those taking dutasteride had a higher incidence of sexual side effects, such as erectile dysfunction (ED) and ejaculatory dysfunction ($P<.01$) compared with those on finasteride.[15] In sum, men presenting with LUTS secondary to BPH on finasteride had less adverse events.

Anticholinergics Therapy

As LUTS secondary to BPH treatment has developed, a new class of drug therapies has emerged known as anticholinergics, once thought to be contraindicated in men suffering from BPH. The use of this pharmacotherapy has been effective in treating detrusor overactivity as well as storage symptoms.[8,16] Drug therapies currently available are MRAs, also known as anticholinergics. There have been limited RCTs assessing direct head-to-head trials evaluating the efficacy of different anticholinergics. In 2008, Kaplan and colleagues[17] evaluated the efficacy of tolterodine, solifenacin, or darifenacin in 107 men with LUTS secondary to BPH currently taking α-blockers with overactive bladder (OAB). The study criteria were defined as men over the age of 45 years, those who had documented micturition frequency more than 8 voids per day, urgency more than 3 times per day, and an IPSS score greater than 12.[17] Kaplan and colleagues[17] evaluated efficacy through evaluating micturitions over a 24-hour period and urgency as well as IPSS scores. Tolterodine, solifenacin, and darifenacin were all effective in reducing frequency over 24 hours and total IPSS scores ($P<.05$).[17] Furthermore, those taking tolterodine ($P<.01$) and solifenacin ($P<.05$) showed significant reductions in micturition frequency and IPSS storage symptoms ($P<.01$).[17] Darifenacin showed a significant increase in overall PVR (≥50 mL).[17] Five individuals taking darifenacin went into urinary retention and required a catheter to alleviate the adverse event.[17] In conclusion, daridenacin was not recommended as an effective line of therapy to improve symptoms of LUTS

secondary to BPH due to the profile of increased side effects.

β-3-Andrenoceptor Agonists

In the bladder, β-3-andrenoceptor agonists are known to be the principal subtype among all β-adrenoceptors.[11] In multiple studies, it has been shown that stimulation of these types of receptors may feasibly increase a patient's bladder capacity without compromising other important urinary factors.[11] β-3-Adrenoceptor agonists are recommended for men with LUTS secondary to BPH with OAB.[11] Globally, there have been several clinical trials evaluating the safety, efficacy, and tolerance among men with LUTS using the β3-agonist mirabegron.[18] Mirabegron targets receptors located on the smooth muscle to decrease detrusor overactivity while promoting relaxation of urothelial functions.[19] Using mirabegron, Nitti and colleagues[20] assessed different urodynamic parameters of men with bladder outlet obstruction and LUTS. In total, 200 men were enrolled in the study with 3 groups: mirabegron 50 mg, mirabegron 100 mg, and a placebo.[20] After a 3-month follow-up, the researchers discovered a significant decrease in urinary frequency versus those taking the placebo,[20] whereas those in the mirabegron 50-mg group showed the most significant decrease in urine urgency. Although results are promising, further studies are needed that evaluate direct head-to-head comparisons to assess this new therapy.

In a systematic literature review, Maman and colleagues[21] compared the efficacy and safety of various medical treatments used to manage symptoms of OAB. In their analysis, they used changes in symptoms such as micturition frequency and incontinence and the incidence of adverse effects that are associated with various OAB medications.[21] They discovered mirabegron was as effective as anticholinergics in reducing frequency of micturition incontinence along with a lower incidence of adverse events.[21]

Phosphodiesterase Type 5 Inhibitors

Despite the main objective to alleviate symptoms of LUTS and BPH, many treatments can cause adverse events, which can be detrimental on the patient's sexual function during and beyond treatment. Because of these adverse effects, the introduction of PDE5-Is has been evaluated and identified as a viable form of treatment to combat LUTS/BPH and comorbidities such as ED.[22] The most commonly used PDE5-Is are sildenafil, tadalafil, and vardenafil. Patients with BPH-LUTS and who have a history of ED are viable candidates for this line of drug treatment.[22] These agents work to increase intracellular levels of cGMP, which in turn reduce detrusor, prostate, and urethra smooth muscle tone.[8] The only significant difference among these drugs is their duration of action with tadalafil lasting up to 32 hours longer than the others.[23] Clinical studies have demonstrated that the use of either of these PDE5-Is can have significant improvements in LUTS in men with BPH.[23] Despite this, clinical trials have not showed any meaningful changes in outlet obstruction such as PVR volume.[23]

Unfortunately, there are no clinical trials assessing the effectiveness of PDE5-Is using direct comparison; however, Yuan and colleagues[24] in their meta-analysis of medical treatments used for LUTS secondary to BPH evaluated the efficacy within the different formulations. The measures evaluated for efficacy were IPSS scores and peak urinary flow rate.[24] Similarly, they found IPSS scores and peak urinary flow were improved comparably across all groups: vardenafil, sildenafil, and tadalafil.[24]

TREATMENT RESISTANCE/COMPLICATIONS

Despite the availability of different pharmacotherapies to alleviate symptoms of LUTS secondary to BPH, there are different adverse events associated with these treatments. α-Blockers represent the most common initial therapy for treating LUTS secondary to BPH. The most common side effects associated with the use of α-blockers are dizziness, rhinitis, and retrograde ejaculation, which are the result of a decline in blood pressure.[25] Clinical studies have shown α-blockers that are uroselective tend to have fewer side effects, but may result in light-headedness and an increased affinity for abnormal ejaculation.[26] Silodosin has favorable cardiovascular tolerability, but a common side effect is abnormal ejaculation, which is defined as retrograde or absence of ejaculation.[8] In 2005, a condition known as floppy iris syndrome was discovered in patients undergoing cataract surgery who had been taking α-blockers.[8]

The PDE5-Is class is a relatively new line of treatment used to treat LUTS secondary to BPH. The most common side effects are headache, dizziness, dyspepsia, and back pain.[26] The contraindication in patients using nitrates, second-generation α-blockers, or antihypertensive medication can increase the severity of these adverse effects.[26] Anticholinergic agents have less severe side effects, which are dry mouth, blurry vision, and constipation.[26,27] Mirabegron, the only β3-agonist available, has been reported to cause "hypertension, headaches, urinary tract infections and nasopharyngitis."[19] Last, those using 5ARIs are prone to have sexual effects, such as a decrease in libido, ED, gynecomastia, and other ejaculatory disorders. In 2 clinical trials, researchers evaluating chemoprevention in prostate cancer found that there is a higher incidence of high-grade cancers in those that are prescribed 5ARIs compared with those in the placebo group.[11]

Patient adherence and compliance are described as drug therapy along with how the patient's attitudes toward taking medications align with the advice received from medical professionals.[28,29] In a study by Cindolo and colleagues,[28] they evaluated patient adherence to monotherapy, combination therapy, and clinical consequences in men with LUTS secondary to BPH. They found that from 6 months to 1 year, patients had an overall 29% adherence, and by 5 years after treatment, adherence had declined further.[28] However, those taking combination therapy treatments were prone to lower adherence than those using monotherapy.[28]

SUMMARY

In conclusion, α-blockers, 5ARIs, anticholinergics, β3-agonists, and PDE5Is are all effective in treating symptoms of LUTS secondary to BPH. In a meta-analysis, Yuan and colleagues[24] found that α-blockers such as doxazosin and terazosin were most effective in improving IPSS and peak urinary flow rate as well as being the least expensive. 5ARIs had significant advantages over other treatments in reducing prostatic volume, prostate cancer, the risk of surgical intervention, and acute urinary retention.[24] MRAs were not able to significantly improve peak urinary flow rate (PUF) or IPSS scores. PDE5Is are the most efficient way of improving ED and were able to improve symptoms of LUTS secondary to BPH, but not PUF.[24] Drug therapies for LUTS secondary to BPH have generally well-received tolerability among patients with mild side effects.

REFERENCES

1. Lepor H. Pathophysiology, epidemiology, and natural history of benign prostatic hyperplasia. Rev Urol 2004;6(Suppl 9):S3–10.
2. Cunningham GR, Kadmon D, O'Leary M, et al. Epidemiology and pathogenesis of benign prostatic

hyperplasia 2015. Available at: http://www.uptodate.com/contents/epidemiology-and-pathogenesis-of-benign-prostatic-hyperplasia.

3. Logie JW, Clifford GM, Farmer RD, et al. Lower urinary tract symptoms suggestive of benign prostatic obstruction–triumph: the role of general practice databases. Eur Urol 2001;39(Suppl 3): 42–7.

4. Wei JT, Calhoun E, Jacobsen SJ. Urologic diseases in America project: benign prostatic hyperplasia. J Urol 2008;179:S75–80.

5. Nickel JC, Mendez-Probst CE, Whelan TF, et al. 2010 Update: guidelines for the management of benign prostatic hyperplasia. Can Urol Assoc J 2010;4:310–6.

6. Oelke M, Bachmann A, Descazeaud A, et al. EAU guidelines on the treatment and follow-up of non-neurogenic male lower urinary tract symptoms including benign prostatic obstruction. Eur Urol 2013;64:118–40.

7. McVary KT, Roehrborn CG, Avins AL, et al. Update on AUA guideline on the management of benign prostatic hyperplasia. J Urol 2011;185:1793–803.

8. Fonseca J, Martins da Silva C. The diagnosis and treatment of lower urinary tract symptoms due to benign prostatic hyperplasia with alpha-blockers: focus on silodosin. Clin Drug Investig 2015; 35(Suppl 1):7–18.

9. Chapple CR, Montorsi F, Tammela TL, et al. Silodosin therapy for lower urinary tract symptoms in men with suspected benign prostatic hyperplasia: results of an international, randomized, double-blind, placebo- and active-controlled clinical trial performed in Europe. Eur Urol 2011;59:342–52.

10. Osman NI, Chapple CR, Cruz F, et al. Silodosin: a new subtype selective alpha-1 antagonist for the treatment of lower urinary tract symptoms in patients with benign prostatic hyperplasia. Expert Opin Pharmacother 2012;13:2085–96.

11. Silva J, Silva CM, Cruz F. Current medical treatment of lower urinary tract symptoms/BPH: do we have a standard? Curr Opin Urol 2014;24:21–8.

12. Robinson D, Garmo H, Holmberg L, et al. 5-alpha reductase inhibitors, benign prostatic hyperplasia, and risk of male breast cancer. Cancer Causes Control 2015;26:1289–97.

13. Kruep EJ, Phillips E, Hogue S, et al. Early symptom improvement and discontinuation of 5-alpha-reductase inhibitor (5ARI) therapy in patients with benign prostatic hyperplasia (BPH). Ann Pharmacother 2014;48:343–8.

14. Nickel JC, Gilling P, Tammela TL, et al. Comparison of dutasteride and finasteride for treating benign prostatic hyperplasia: the Enlarged Prostate International Comparator Study (EPICS). BJU Int 2011;108: 388–94.

15. Kaplan SA, Chung DE, Lee RK, et al. A 5-year retrospective analysis of 5alpha-reductase inhibitors in men with benign prostatic hyperplasia: finasteride has comparable urinary symptom efficacy and prostate volume reduction, but less sexual side effects and breast complications than dutasteride. Int J Clin Pract 2012;66: 1052–5.

16. Abrams P, Kaplan S, De Koning Gans HJ, et al. Safety and tolerability of tolterodine for the treatment of overactive bladder in men with bladder outlet obstruction. J Urol 2006;175:999–1004 [discussion: 1004].

17. Kaplan SA, Zoltan E, Te AE. Saftey and efficacy of tolterodine, solifenacin, and darifenacin in men with lower urinary tract symptoms (LUTS) on alpha-blockers with persistent overactive bladder symptoms (OAB). J Urol 2008;179:701.

18. Khullar V, Amarenco G, Angulo JC, et al. Efficacy and tolerability of mirabegron, a beta(3)-adrenoceptor agonist, in patients with overactive bladder: results from a randomised European-Australian phase 3 trial. Eur Urol 2013;63:283–95.

19. Sacco E, Bientinesi R. Mirabegron: a review of recent data and its prospects in the management of overactive bladder. Ther Adv Urol 2012;4: 315–24.

20. Nitti VW, Rosenberg S, Mitcheson DH, et al. Urodynamics and safety of the beta(3)-adrenoceptor agonist mirabegron in males with lower urinary tract symptoms and bladder outlet obstruction. J Urol 2013;190:1320–7.

21. Maman K, Aballea S, Nazir J, et al. Comparative efficacy and safety of medical treatments for the management of overactive bladder: a systematic literature review and mixed treatment comparison. Eur Urol 2014;65:755–65.

22. Miller MS. Role of phosphodiesterase type 5 inhibitors for lower urinary tract symptoms. Ann Pharmacother 2013;47:278–83.

23. Lepor H. Medical treatment of benign prostatic hyperplasia. Rev Urol 2011;13:20–33.

24. Yuan JQ, Mao C, Wong SY, et al. Comparative effectiveness and safety of monodrug therapies for lower urinary tract symptoms associated with benign prostatic hyperplasia: a network meta-analysis. Medicine (Baltimore) 2015;94:e974.

25. Lepor H, Kazzazi A, Djavan B. alpha-Blockers for benign prostatic hyperplasia: the new era. Curr Opin Urol 2012;22:7–15.

26. Rosenberg MT, Staskin D, Riley J, et al. The evaluation and treatment of prostate-related LUTS in the primary care setting: the next STEP. Curr Urol Rep 2013;14:595–605.

27. Rosenberg MT, Staskin DR, Kaplan SA, et al. A practical guide to the evaluation and treatment

of male lower urinary tract symptoms in the primary care setting. Int J Clin Pract 2007;61: 1535–46.

28. Cindolo L, Pirozzi L, Sountoulides P, et al. Patient's adherence on pharmacological therapy for benign prostatic hyperplasia (BPH)-associated lower urinary tract symptoms (LUTS) is different: is combination therapy better than monotherapy? BMC Urol 2015;15:96.

29. Cindolo L, Pirozzi L, Fanizza C, et al. Drug adherence and clinical outcomes for patients under pharmacological therapy for lower urinary tract symptoms related to benign prostatic hyperplasia: population-based cohort study. Eur Urol 2015;68:418–25.

Prostatic Urethral Lift
A Unique Minimally Invasive Surgical Treatment of Male Lower Urinary Tract Symptoms Secondary to Benign Prostatic Hyperplasia

Claus G. Roehrborn, MD

KEYWORDS

- Prostatic urethral lift • Benign prostatic hyperplasia • Lower urinary tract symptoms
- Sexual function • Minimally invasive therapy • Surgical therapy

KEY POINTS

- Prostatic urethral lift can be performed in the office with local anesthesia.
- Return to normalcy is rapid, typically without a catheter.
- Symptom improvement is rapid, significant, and sustained to at least 4 years.
- Sexual function is preserved.
- Future treatment options for patients are preserved.

INTRODUCTION: NATURE OF THE PROBLEM

Traditional treatment options for male lower urinary tract symptoms (LUTS) due to benign prostatic hyperplasia (BPH) include watchful waiting with lifestyle management, medical therapy, and interventional procedures. Each approach is associated with positive and negative attributes and represents an important tool for the practicing urologist. Despite the number and variety of approaches, there still exists a large population of men who are underserved by these standard options and desire a therapy that has fewer side effects and offers faster recovery compared with standard surgery, yet is more effective and less burdensome than lifelong medical therapy.

Shortcomings of traditional therapies limit the population of patients to which they can be applied. The least disruptive of the treatment approaches is watchful waiting with lifestyle management. Although this approach exposes patients to minimal iatrogenic risk, it is generally limited to patients with mild or moderate symptom frequency and severity and low bother due to the symptoms. Medications are associated with modest symptom relief (3.5–7.5 International Prostate Symptom Score [IPSS] improvement compared with 0–5.7 for placebo) but carry the burden of daily, lifetime dosing and not insignificant side effects.[1] As many as 25% of men on drug therapy are dissatisfied and discontinue treatment.[2] The most invasive treatment option is surgical therapy, whereby tissue is removed either by transurethral resection of the prostate (TURP) or ablative laser procedures (vaporization or enucleation). TURP, the gold standard surgery, results in 14.9 IPSS improvement at 1 year.[1] This substantial improvement in symptoms can be associated with significant postoperative morbidity, however, as complications from TURP include urinary incontinence (3%), urethral stricture (7%), erectile dysfunction (10%), and

Department of Urology, UT Southwestern Medical Center, 5323 Harry Hines Boulevard, J8 142, Dallas, TX 75390-9110, USA
E-mail address: Claus.roehrborn@utsouthwestern.edu

Urol Clin N Am 43 (2016) 357–369
http://dx.doi.org/10.1016/j.ucl.2016.04.008
0094-0143/16/$ – see front matter

ejaculatory dysfunction (65%).[1,3] Catheterization after TURP is expected, and patients are counseled to expect 4 to 6 weeks of worsened irritative symptoms. Laser therapy demonstrates superior control of bleeding to TURP but is similar in effectiveness, anesthesia requirement, and complication rates.[4]

Existing minimally invasive thermotherapies such as transurethral microwave therapy (TUMT), transurethral needle ablation (TUNA), and steam injection (REZUM) induce tissue damage and necrosis by different heat sources. Their effectiveness is superior to medications but inferior to TURP (10.2 and 9.1 point improvement in IPSS at 1 year for TUMT and TUNA, respectively).[1] Because of the thermal injury, there is a healing response, tissue inflammation, and irritative voiding symptoms in most patients during the first few months after treatment.[1] After the procedure, patients experience routine catheterization, a 20% to 25% risk of acute urinary retention, and irritative voiding symptoms that last for 4 to 6 weeks.[1,5] The 3 TUMT patient groups in the Coretherm pivotal study underwent 14, 18, and 20 days mean posttreatment indwelling catheter time.[6] Further, TUMT therapies have been associated with a greater than 20% retrograde ejaculation rate.[7,8] Lower power alternatives were developed to minimize adverse effects, but effectiveness was greatly compromised as well. Retreatment rates for thermal ablation techniques have been disappointing, reaching as high as 20% to 50% by 3 years.[9] Because of limitations with the technologies and the difficult patient experience after the procedure, the number of minimally invasive thermotherapy procedures among Medicare beneficiaries increased gradually to modest levels of 37,637 in 2005 and then have precipitously declined.[10,11]

The prostatic urethral lift (PUL) is a nonthermal technology to treat patients who want superior efficacy with minimal risk. With the high prevalence of patients who discontinue medications and the declining number who pursue surgical or minimally invasive therapy, there is a significant population of suffering men who are inadequately treated by the currently available treatment options. The PUL procedure uses a mechanical approach, and the mechanism of action is to pin the lateral lobes out of the way and thereby reduce obstruction. By not requiring biological response to tissue removal or thermal injury, PUL can offer a more rapid recovery, freedom from urinary catheterization, and the opportunity to achieve significant symptom relief with low morbidity.

SURGICAL TECHNIQUE
Preoperative Planning

Selecting the most appropriate LUTS therapy for any patient requires careful consideration of the patients' history, condition, risk tolerance, and desired outcome. Because BPH is a quality-of-life issue, it is important to understand how symptom relief, perioperative experience, sexual function preservation, and continence preservation contribute to the overall outcome for a specific patient; if a man achieves LUTS relief yet loses the ability to perform sexually or maintain continence, his quality of life (QoL) may not be improved. The PUL procedure has been shown to improve QoL by improving LUTS while offering more rapid recovery without compromising sexual function or continence.[12,13]

Proper patient selection among patients who desire the therapy is a key component to ensuring the best clinical outcome. Typically, patients have a prostate volume less than 80 mL, when not on medical therapy an IPSS greater than 12 with associated bother, and Qmax (peak flow rate) less than 15 mL/s. Baseline prostate volume and prostate length have not been found to be predictors of symptom response.[9] It is important to note that a large portion of the clinical data involves patients who are washed out of any BPH medication, and baseline symptoms of medicated patients might be somewhat lower. Although definitive data on patients with large prostates are lacking, patients have been treated with prostates up to 145 mL.[14,15] Patients in active urinary retention or on anticoagulation have not been studied and, therefore, should be approached with caution. Patients should be instructed to discontinue anticoagulants before the procedure in collaboration with their prescribing provider. At present, direct PUL treatment of the obstructive median lobe is being studied and is currently contraindicated in the USA [ClinicalTrials.gov Identifier: NCT02625545]. As all BPH patients have a median lobe to one extent or another, it is important to assess cystoscopically whether lateral lobe opening would be sufficient. **Fig. 1**A shows an obstructive median lobe that would likely not be effectively addressed with simple lateral lobe pinning; **Fig. 1**B shows a median lobe that, although protruding, offers enough space anteriorly to not pose an issue for standard lateral lobe UroLift.

In order to determine whether a patient is an ideal candidate, the target locations and number of implants, and the ability to perform the procedure in the clinic, a planning cystoscopy and transrectal ultrasound (TRUS) are useful. The author often performs TRUS to determine prostate volume, presence and size of a median lobe, and to aid in procedure planning. In addition to its

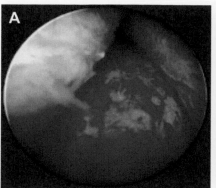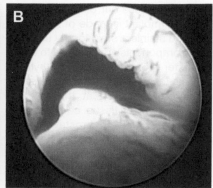

Fig. 1. An obstructive median lobe that would likely not be addressed with lateral lobe PUL (*A*); a protruding median lobe that offers enough space anteriorly to be addressed with lateral lobe implants only (*B*).

obvious diagnostic utility, flexible cystoscopy is helpful in determining patient tolerance to a local anesthesia–based UroLift procedure. Patients who tolerate flexible cystoscopy in the clinic have an increased likelihood of having a positive office-based PUL treatment experience.[16]

Preparation and Patient Positioning

The procedure may be conducted in the clinic, ambulatory surgery center, or operating room. The primary determinant for venue selection may be anesthesia considerations. The procedure may be performed under general, spinal, regional, or local anesthesia with oral or intravenous sedation.[12,16] In the LIFT (Luminal Improvement Following Prostatic Tissue Approximation for the Treatment of Lower Urinary Tract Symptoms) study, all but one of the subjects treated in North America received local anesthesia (4 patients had a periprostatic block).[12] Approaches to local anesthesia include oral sedatives, such as diazepam, administered 30 minutes before the procedure. Typical local anesthetic regimen calls for 18F floppy catheter bladder drainage followed by injection of cold lidocaine liquid into the bladder and cold lidocaine gel into the urethra. The penis is then clamped for 20 minutes with patients recumbent. Patients

who are given minimal anesthesia may be counseled before the procedure to expect some discomfort when the rigid cystoscope traverses the bladder neck. A bedside nurse and intraoperative physician narrative during the procedure have been found to be helpful for conscious patients.[17]

The procedure room should be arranged for a transurethral procedure with patients placed in the lithotomy position and the cystoscopic monitor positioned for direct visualization. The PUL system telescope requires a 2.9-mm, 0° lens, and 20F cystoscopy sheath with custom bridge (**Fig. 2**A). This reusable scope kit can be acquired from either Storz or NeoTract, the provider of UroLift implants. The PUL implants are preloaded in the UroLift system delivery devices; typically 4 implants are placed and should be brought into the room in advance. Antibiotic prophylaxis is left to the discretion of the treating surgeon and local policies.

Surgical Approach

The surgical goal is to deobstruct urine outflow from the bladder by creating an open, continuous channel through the anterior aspect of the prostatic urethra from the bladder neck to the verumontanum. The channel is shaped by placing small, permanent, metallic UroLift implants into

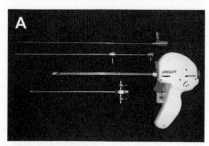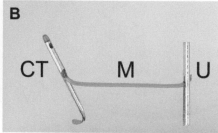

Fig. 2. UroLift system and associated equipment: (*A*) UroLift delivery device with 2.9-mm telescope, 20F sheath, and visual obturator; (*B*) UroLift implant composed of capsular tab (CT), polyester monofilament (M), and urethral endpiece (U). (*Courtesy of* NeoTract, Pleasanton, CA; with permission.)

the prostate to lift the tissue out of the way (see **Fig. 2**B). The UroLift implant is made of nitinol for the capsular tab and stainless steel for the urethral endpiece. These components are tethered to each other via a polyester monofilament (polyethylene terephthalate), the length of which is adjusted automatically by the instrument at the time of deployment. The amount of tissue compression and, hence, the opening of the prostatic fossa are determined by the surgeon manually deflecting the prostate lobe using the rigid instrument. The delivered implant then functions to hold that extent of compression in place as the tissue remodels over time.

UroLift implants are placed in the lateral direction and are usually paired with one implant on the left and one implant on the right. The first pair is placed approximately 1.5 cm distal to the bladder neck in order to open the proximal aspect of the prostate while ensuring that no component is deployed onto the bladder neck or into the bladder mucosa. After placement of implants on both sides in the proximal urethra, the resulting channel is assessed with a cystoscope, typically with the 2.9-mm telescope and special bridge. Most often an additional pair of implants is placed just anterior to the verumontanum to maximize the caliber and length of the channel (**Fig. 3**). Depending on morphology and tissue compliance, additional implants may be needed to adequately reshape the urethra. No significant correlations have been found between the number of implants placed during the procedure and symptom response afterwards.[9] In the LIFT randomized study, the median number of implants was 4, whereas the mean was 4.9.[12] Eighty-six percent of procedures required 6 or less implants for prostates ranging from 30 to 77 cm^3.

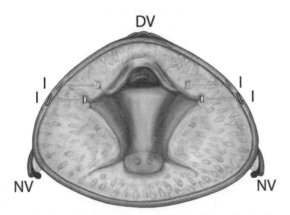

Fig. 3. The PUL procedure. Implants (I) reside in the anterolateral prostate, below the dorsal venous complex (DV) and anterior to the neurovascular bundles (NV).

Surgical Procedure

After insertion of the 20F cystoscope to the bladder, the telescope/bridge is replaced with the UroLift delivery device housing the 2.9-mm telescope. Postoperative adverse effects can be minimized by careful technique throughout the procedure and reducing the amount of tissue manipulation and mucosal trauma. Before retracting the device from bladder to prostate, the device is rotated such that the needle exit port is pointed laterally in the direction of the first target location. The delivery device is then withdrawn such that the tip of the device enters the prostatic urethra approximately 1.5 cm distal to the bladder neck. Using the external urethral sphincter as the pivot point, the delivery device is pivoted approximately 20° to 30° laterally such that the prostate tissue is compressed. Because the anterior aspect of the urethra is of primary importance, the point of compression should preferentially treat that portion of the urethra with one-third of the tissue anterior and two-thirds posterior to the target location.

Once the target tissue is compressed, the implant is delivered through a series of triggers (**Fig. 4**). First, the safety lock is released. Second, squeezing the blue needle trigger rapidly advances the hollow 19-Ga needle. At this point, a portion of the needle body is visible cystoscopically at the tip of the device. Third, retracting both the blue and gray triggers together retracts the needle, unsheathing the implant; the suture, which can now be seen cystoscopically, is then automatically tensioned at the end of retraction. Tensioning the suture ensures that the capsular component is pulled down onto the fibromuscular capsule, and suture length is sized to the compressed width of the prostate lobe. Fourth, the device is then moved 1 to 3 mm proximally until light reflection is seen on the suture (**Fig. 5**); then depressing the blue release button installs the urethral component and severs excess suture.

Once implants have been placed into the right and left sides proximally, the resulting channel should be assessed cystoscopically from the verumontanum. Additional implants may be required. If so, they should be placed just anterior to the verumontanum, again in the top one-third of the prostate, so as to open the apical prostatic fossa. Occasionally, after apical implants, a continuous anterior channel is not observed from verumontanum to bladder neck; additional midprostate implants may be required. A unique aspect of the PUL procedure is that the goal is to develop a continuous channel through the anterior aspect of the prostatic fossa. As can be seen in

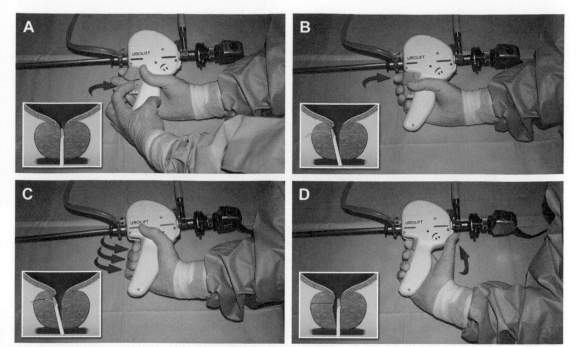

Fig. 4. UroLift implant delivery steps: (*A*) release safety mechanism; (*B*) deploy needle; (*C*) retract needle and deliver monofilament tension; and (*D*) secure urethral endpiece and cut monofilament. (*Courtesy of* NeoTract, Pleasanton, CA; with permission.)

Fig. 6, often in larger prostates the bulk of prostate tissue, located posterolaterally, is not affected. The reason to preferentially address the anterior is that further sculpting of the posterior tissue could cause tissue to encroach on the anterior channel. Early investigations showed better results when addressing a single anterior channel,[15] and this has been the established method in later studies.[12,16]

Mean treatment time ranged from 52 to 66 minutes in the US clinical trials, which included each investigator's very first procedures.[12,16] After a typical learning curve of 10 to 15 cases, procedure time decreases substantially Although postprocedure imaging is not necessary or routine, initial studies used fluoroscopy to confirm that the capsular component could be repeatedly placed on the capsular surface or pubic fascia.[14,15,17] Computed tomography (CT) scans have also been used to demonstrate final implant location with respect to surrounding structures and confirm that the implants remain far from critical structures (**Fig. 7**A). The implants are tested and rated as MRI compatible. A small periurethral artifact can be seen on MRI because of the stainless steel urethral component (see **Fig. 7**B). As the remainder of the prostate is free from artifact, MRI-guided diagnostic and treatment options remain feasible.

Immediate Postoperative Care

Immediate care after the procedure depends on anesthesia selection. Although patients treated under general anesthesia need to be monitored in the recovery room, most patients with regional

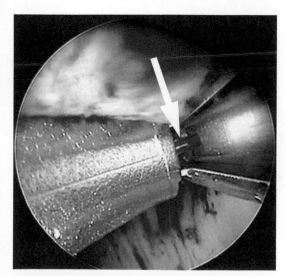

Fig. 5. After needle retraction, the delivery device is advanced toward bladder 3 to 4 mm until a reflection (*arrow*) is seen on the monofilament. At this point the urethral endpiece can be delivered.

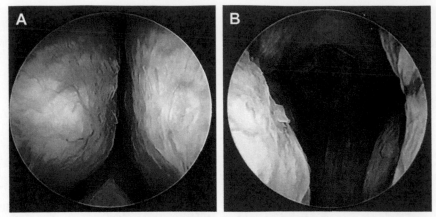

Fig. 6. Baseline cystoscopy shows kissing lateral lobes (*A*). After PUL, implants have opened the prostatic fossa (*B*). Note that apical lateral lobe tissue is less addressed than the anterior prostatic fossa.

or local anesthetic can be sent home without delay.[16] Depending on the amount of hematuria, some patients may require an overnight catheter. As the urologist develops proficiency with the technique, he or she can better avoid mucosal abrasion and the need for postoperative catheterization is reduced. Overnight catheterization decreased from 32% of void-tested patients in the original US study to 20% in the follow-on study, and lower rates are likely achievable by experienced users.[12,16] Mean catheter duration of the entire cohort was less than a day in the US studies.[12,16]

Postoperative adverse effects are similar to rigid cystoscopy: mild to moderate hematuria, dysuria, urgency, urge incontinence, and pelvic discomfort. These issues have been shown to typically resolve within 2 weeks, and it is prudent to advise patients to expect them at some level for 2 to 4 weeks. Many patients are free of adverse effects within days; mean return to normal activity is 5 to

8 days, depending on the study.[12,16] Postoperative pelvic discomfort is typically managed with ibuprofen. For patients less tolerant of dysuria, phenazopyridine hydrochloride has been effective; for those intolerant of postoperative urgency, anticholinergic agents may be helpful. Typically neither of these pharmaceuticals is required. Although the clinical studies typically required medication washout, in standard practice patients are usually on an alpha-blocker or combination therapy and can be counseled to continue treatment for 2 weeks postoperatively particularly with an alpha-blocker and then discontinue medication.

REHABILITATION AND RECOVERY

Because the PUL approach is mechanical and does not rely on recovery from tissue removal or thermal injury, patients have a fast recovery. Recovery may last weeks to months after a traditional

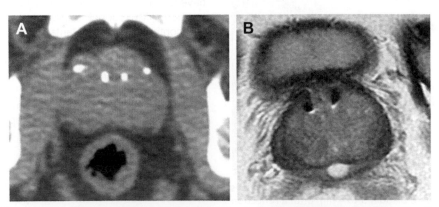

Fig. 7. UroLift implants within prostate as seen via CT radiograph (*A*) and MRI (*B*). A small periurethral artifact is seen on MRI.

surgery, such as TURP, and is burdensome for patients and their families.[18] In a European multicenter randomized comparison between PUL and TURP, recovery experience was compared via a quality-of-recovery visual analog scale (QoR VAS). The number of subjects reporting high-quality recovery as defined as QoR VAS of 70% or greater by 1 month was considerably greater for PUL than for TURP (82% vs 53%, $P<.01$).[13] The time course thereafter is particularly interesting, at recovery in the TURP cohort only caught up to the PUL cohort between 6 and 12 months (**Fig. 8**).[13] Further, patient satisfaction increased more quickly for PUL than for TURP.[13] In a separate study conducted in the United States, 86.3% of PUL subjects achieved QoR VAS of 80% or greater by 1 month.[16]

Disruption to the patients' lives due to the procedure is minimal. On average, patients have been found to return to preoperative activity in 5.1 days and return to work in less than 3 days.[16] At 1 month, the percentage of work missed as assessed by the Work Productivity and Activity Impairment questionnaire was 0%, with only 3% overall work impairment reported.[16] LUTS also respond quickly to the procedure, demonstrating between 4.1 and 8.1 average IPSS improvement by 2 weeks.[12,14,16] At 1 month, 90% of patients report improvement via the Patient Global Impression of Improvement index and 75% of subjects would recommend the procedure to a relative or friend.[16]

CLINICAL RESULTS IN THE LITERATURE

Several clinical studies since 2005 have established the safety and effectiveness of the PUL procedure. Two trials were multinational, prospective, randomized studies. The first randomized trial was the LIFT study for Food and Drug (FDA) clearance that randomized subjects to control (sham) or PUL procedure. Level 1b evidence was achieved by incorporating a double blind of patient and assessor during the randomized comparison. The BPH6 study was a randomized comparison between PUL and TURP in a cohort restricted to a prostate size less than 60 cm³. This study compared the two cohorts via traditional measures as well as through a composite end point (BPH6) derived from portions of previously validated questionaires.[13] Other notable studies include the feasibility study that documented first-in-man experience, the LOCAL (UroLift System TOlerability and ReCovery When Administering Local Anesthesia) trial that assessed patients for early outcomes, and the crossover study that followed the LIFT study control patients after crossover to active PUL therapy.[9,14–16,19]

Studies on the PUL procedure have been conducted in the United States, Canada, Europe, and Australia. Patient inclusion and exclusion criteria were relatively consistent between the large trials, with patients 50 years old or older, IPSS greater than 12, and Qmax less than 12 to 15 mL/s. Prostate volume ranges have varied, with the US studies ranging from 30 to 80 cm³ and European and Australian studies typically ranging up to 100 cm³.[9,14–17,19] The BPH6 study limited prostate size to 60 cm³. Exclusion criteria included previous pelvic procedure, obstructive median lobe, active urinary tract infection, current urinary retention, prostate-specific antigen greater than 10 ng/mL unless normal biopsy, and inability to give informed consent. Follow-up assessments were conducted at regular intervals and included the IPSS, IPSS QoL, BPH Impact Index (BPHII), peak flow rate (Qmax), postvoid residual volume (PVR), Sexual Health Inventory for Men (SHIM), and Male Sexual Health Questionnaire for Ejaculatory Dysfunction (MSHQ-EjD). **Table 1** details the patient demographics of the largest clinical trials.

Effectiveness

Symptom response has been shown to occur as rapidly as 2 weeks after the procedure and remains durable for at least 4 years (**Fig. 9**, **Table 2**). The LOCAL study focused on perioperative and early outcomes, including IPSS, QoL, BPHII, and peak flow rate (Qmax) change. Patients demonstrated significant early improvement in their symptoms, with 5.7 (24%) and 10.5 (48%) IPSS improvement at 2 weeks and 1 month, respectively.[16] QoL improved in a parallel manner, with 1.7 (33%) and 2.1 (44%) improvement at 2 weeks and 1 month. The impact of BPH on patients followed the symptom response, with patients experiencing 3.4 (45%) improvement in the BPH Impact

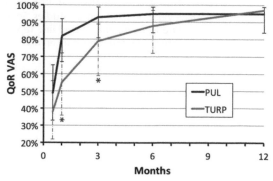

Fig. 8. Percentage of BPH6 randomized study subjects achieving high-quality recovery (≥70% on the QoR VAS) after PUL and TURP (mean, 95% confidence interval). *$P<.05$.

Table 1
Patient demographics in the largest prostatic urethral lift clinical studies

	Feasibility[14,15]	LIFT[9,12]	Crossover[19]	BPH6[13]	LOCAL[16]
Mean (SD)					
Number of patients	64	137	51	44	51
Patient age (y)	67 (7.3)	67 (8.5)	64 (7.8)	64 (7.1)	65 (7.6)
Prostate volume (cm³)	50.8 (23.0)	44.6 (12.5)	40.5 (9.9)	37.8 (11.6)	41.0 (11.6)
Anesthesia time (min)	66.6 (23.0)	52.4 (22.1)	41.1 (12.2)	42.6 (14.4)	48.9 (1512)
Average number of implants	3.9	4.9	4.4	4.7	3.7
Functional scores at baseline					
IPSS	22.9 (5.4)	22.3 (5.5)	25.4 (5.5)	22.1 (5.7)	21.5 (5.4)
QoL	4.9 (0.9)	4.6 (1.1)	4.8 (1.1)	4.6 (1.1)	4.6 (1.0)
BPHII	7.3 (3.0)	6.9 (2.8)	7.3 (3.1)	7.3 (2.5)	6.7 (3.1)
Qmax (mL/s)	8.7 (3.1)	7.9 (2.5)	8.0 (2.4)	10.6 (3.0)	8.0 (2.2)
PVR (mL)	114.8 (103.3)	85.9 (69.0)	88.1 (70.4)	85.9 (71.6)	77.0 (74.9)
SHIM³	11.7 (8.6)	15.9 (7.1)	16.3 (6.7)	19.5 (4.9)	16.5 (7.3)
MSHQ-EjD Function	8.9 (3.9)	8.7 (3.2)	8.8 (3.0)	10.5 (2.7)	10.0 (2.3)
MSHQ-EjD Bother	1.7 (1.5)	2.3 (1.6)	2.2 (1.7)	1.7 (1.8)	2.0 (1.3)

Index by 1 month. Peak flow rate was likewise affected, with 3.3 mL/s (47%) improvement by 1 month. Similar early outcomes by 2 and 4 weeks were seen in all other studies.

After the initial rapid response during the first month, symptoms continue to improve through 3 months. Patients experienced between 11.1 and 13.6 IPSS improvement (48%–60% change) at 3 months.[12–15,17] Subjects in the LIFT randomized study have recently completed the 4-year follow-up, which further demonstrates the stability of the response. Matched paired data show a 40% to 45% improvement in IPSS at years 1 through 4 (**Table 3**). QoL and BPH Impact Index response follow the changes in IPSS, with 4-year

improvements for QoL at 2.4 points (52%) and BPHII at 3.7 points (54%). Peak flow rate (Qmax) improvement through 4 years remained stable, with 4.0 mL/s, 4.2 mL/s, 3.5 mL/s, and 4.2 mL/s improvement at 1, 2, 3, and 4 years, respectively.

It is important to appreciate the quality of the LIFT randomized study when qualifying the data. Of the 140 patients in the UroLift treated arm, 11 (8%) discontinued the study, 3 (2%) relocated away from the study site, and 8 (6%) missed the 4-year visit. Additionally, 6 (4%) patients died of unrelated causes and 4 (3%) exited the study because of unrelated cancers. Although 108 (77%) patients were available for follow-up, data from 29 were excluded from analysis because of either BPH

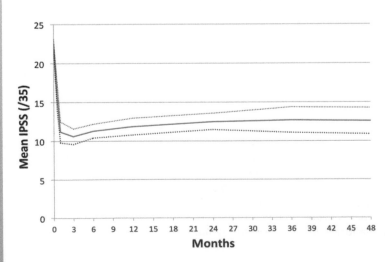

Fig. 9. Meta-analysis of IPSS over 4 years across 4 clinical studies. Solid line is mean, and dotted line represents 95% confidence interval.

Table 2
Calculated composite International Prostate Symptom Score after prostatic urethral lift from 4 large published studies with 95% confidence intervals

Months	0	0.5	1	3	6	12	24	36	48
Mean	22.5	15.8	11.2	10.6	11.3	11.9	12.5	12.7	12.6
95% Confidence Interval Bounds									
Lower	21.8	13.9	9.8	9.6	10.4	10.8	11.5	11.1	10.9
Upper	23.1	17.6	12.5	11.6	12.2	13.0	13.6	14.4	14.3

retreatment or protocol deviation. This censoring provides more scientifically valid data for **Table 3**, yet the question can be asked as to how different the data might look if all were included. Analyzing the pooled population of 108 subjects (108 of 140, 77%) with follow-up data 4 years after the index PUL procedure, the improvements from baseline at 4 years in IPSS (8.7), QoL (2.3), BPH II (3.6), and Qmax (5.1) were similar to the original paired analysis after incorporating the censored subjects (see **Table 3**). A comparison between the changes experienced by censored subjects and the rest of the cohort resulted in P values that ranged from .12 to .76 and indicated a lack of statistical bias in censoring these subjects.

Reviewing pivotal data from other BPH therapies sets the aforementioned LIFT study quality into context. The percentage of LIFT subjects without data at 4 years (23%) is similar to the 18% TURP subjects missing in the 3-year Veterans Affairs Cooperative Study on TURP.[20] Of the 51 subjects (51 of 280, 18%) with no data, 24 had been withdrawn, 13 died of unrelated causes, and 14 were lost to follow-up.[20]

Minimally invasive treatment trials reported patients lost for follow-up in 30%,[21] 35%,[22] or even 62% at 4 years.[23]

It has been well established that removal of prostate tissue (simple prostatectomy, TURP, laser, and so forth) offers maximal improvements on urinary symptoms and flow. A common goal in less invasive therapies is to offer adequate symptom and flow improvements while avoiding the unwanted negative effects of surgery. To quantify this goal, the BPH6 composite end point was developed. This end point has yet to be validated but nonetheless offers a valuable, if preliminary, method by which to compare treatment choices. The BPH6 responder end point, which was used to compare PUL with TURP, incorporated patient-centered treatment goals of (1) adequate symptom relief (IPSS change ≥30%), (2) high-quality recovery (QoR VAS ≥70%), (3) maintenance of erectile function (SHIM reduced <6), (4) maintenance of ejaculatory function (MSHQ, Q3>0), (5) maintenance of continence

(incontinence severity index [ISI] <5), and (6) avoidance of high-grade complications (Clavien-Dindo II+).[13] At 1 year and throughout the follow-up, the number of patients who met the BPH6 end point was significantly higher for PUL over TURP (P = .005).[13]

Safety

Adverse effects of treatment seem to be mild to moderate and consist primarily of transient events. The most commonly reported events in the large studies are mild to moderate hematuria (26%–80%), dysuria (36%–74%), irritative symptoms/discomfort (21%–52%), urinary tract infection (7%–11%), urinary retention (9%), and urge incontinence (2%–8%). Most of these events resolve within 2 to 4 weeks without long-term clinical sequela. New-onset stress urinary incontinence and bleeding requiring transfusion have not been reported in any study.

Encrustation and stone formation are a concern with any foreign body implantation. The large FDA-overseen randomized study required independent review of flexible cystoscopy videos taken at 1 year specifically including retroflexion of the cystoscopes. No UroLift implants were found to encrust when delivered properly within the prostatic fossa. When implants were placed at the bladder neck and exposed to urine in the bladder, however, the components were more likely to encrust. Of the 642 implants reviewed during the LIFT study at 1 year, 14 implants (2%) in 10 subjects were encrusted.[12] Removal of these implants has been achieved through standard transurethral procedures or managed conservatively with monitoring.[9] This important information has led to a change in the technique to assure that the proximal implants are delivered 1.5 cm distal to the bladder neck with the device angled at least 20° to 30° laterally. If an implant is deployed inadvertently such that it protrudes into the bladder, it is prudent to remove it during the index procedure with simple endoscopic forceps graspers. The urethral component is shaped like a clip and can be slid off of the monofilament with routine technique.

Table 3
Paired outcome measures after prostatic urethral lift

Outcome		3 mo	1 y	2 y	3 y	4 y
IPSS	N (Paired)	136	123	103	93	79
	Baseline	22.3 ± 5.5	22.1 ± 5.6	21.8 ± 5.6	21.6 ± 5.9	21.4 ± 5.9
	Follow-up	11.2 ± 7.7	11.5 ± 7.3	12.7 ± 7.9	12.7 ± 7.6	12.6 ± 7.8
	Change	−11.1	−10.6	−9.1	−8.8	−8.8
	% Change (95% CI)	−50% (−55% to −44%)	−47% (−53% to −42%)	−41% (−48% to −35%)	−41% (−48% to −34%)	−41% (−49% to −33%)
	P value	<.0001	<.0001	<.0001	<.0001	<.0001
QoL	N (Paired)	136	123	103	93	79
	Baseline	4.6 ± 1.1	4.6 ± 1.0	4.5 ± 1.0	4.5 ± 1.0	4.5 ± 1.0
	Follow-up	2.4 ± 1.7	2.3 ± 1.6	2.3 ± 1.6	2.2 ± 1.6	2.1 ± 1.4
	Change	−2.2	−2.3	−2.2	−2.3	−2.4
	% Change (95% CI)	−47% (−53% to −40%)	−51% (−57% to −44%)	−47% (−55% to −40%)	−49% (−57% to −41%)	−52% (−60% to −44%)
	P value	<.0001	<.0001	<.0001	<.0001	<.0001
BPHII	N (Paired)	136	123	103	93	79
	Baseline	6.9 ± 2.8	6.8 ± 2.8	6.5 ± 2.9	6.4 ± 2.9	6.3 ± 2.7
	Follow-up	2.9 ± 3.0	2.8 ± 2.9	2.8 ± 3.0	2.7 ± 2.8	2.6 ± 2.6
	Change	−4.0	−4.0	−3.8	−3.8	−3.7
	% Change (95% CI)	−56% (−64% to −48%)	−57% (−66% to −49%)	−55% (−65% to −45%)	−53% (−66% to −41%)	−54% (−65% to −43%)
	P value	<.0001	<.0001	<.0001	<.0001	<.0001
Qmax	N (Paired)	122	102	86	69	61
	Baseline	8.0 ± 2.4	8.0 ± 2.4	8.3 ± 2.4	8.3 ± 2.4	8.4 ± 2.4
	Follow-up	12.3 ± 5.3	12.1 ± 5.3	12.5 ± 5.4	11.8 ± 5.0	12.6 ± 5.6
	Change	4.3	4.0	4.2	3.5	4.2
	% Change (95% CI)	64% (50%–79%)	59% (43%–74%)	59% (41%–77%)	53% (33%–74%)	62% (38%–86%)
	P value	<.0001	<.0001	<.0001	<.0001	<.0001
SHIM	N (Paired)	91	87	72	66	55
	Baseline	16.2 ± 7.0	16.0 ± 7.1	15.6 ± 7.0	16.5 ± 6.8	17.0 ± 6.5
	Follow-up	17.4 ± 7.6	16.7 ± 7.8	16.7 ± 7.6	17.0 ± 7.9	17.3 ± 7.1
	Change	1.3	0.7	1.1	0.5	0.3
	% Change (95% CI)	14% (6%–23%)	19% (−4% to 41%)	22% (−3% to 47%)	4% (−6% to 14%)	7% (−7% to 22%)
	P value	.0041	.2877	.0419	.3306	.4749
MSHQ-Ejd	N (Paired)	91	87	72	66	56
	Baseline	8.7 ± 3.1	8.7 ± 3.3	8.8 ± 3.4	9.2 ± 3.0	9.3 ± 3.1
	Follow-up	11.0 ± 3.2	10.3 ± 3.2	9.8 ± 3.3	9.7 ± 3.5	10.1 ± 3.4
	Change	2.3 ± 2.6	1.6 ± 2.7	1.1 ± 2.5	0.6 ± 2.5	0.8 ± 2.4
	% Change (95% CI)	36% (25%–47%)	28% (17%–38%)	30% (8%–53%)	9% (−1% to 18%)	12% (1%–23%)
	P value	<.0001	<.0001	<.0001	.0128	.0025
MSHQ-Bother	N (Paired)	91	87	72	66	56
	Baseline	2.2 ± 1.7	2.2 ± 1.7	2.3 ± 1.7	2.2 ± 1.6	2.2 ± 1.7
	Follow-up	1.1 ± 1.3	1.4 ± 1.4	1.6 ± 1.5	1.6 ± 1.5	1.3 ± 1.3
	Change	−1.1 ± 1.4	−0.8 ± 1.6	−0.6 ± 1.5	−0.6 ± 1.5	−0.8 ± 1.6
	% Change (95% CI)	−48% (−62% to −33%)	−28% (−45% to −11%)	−21% (−41% to −1%)	−27% (−44% to −11%)	−31% (−50% to −13%)
	P value	<.0001	<.0001	<.0001	.0002	<.0001

Abbreviation: CI, confidence interval.

Sexual Function Preservation

There is no evidence in the literature of degradation in erectile or ejaculatory function after PUL.

As determined by adverse-event collection and adjudicated by an independent clinical events committee, no patient in the FDA randomized study experienced new-onset, sustained erectile or ejaculatory dysfunction.[9,12] Sexual function in this study was also further analyzed in detail and with a groundbreaking methodology.[24] Ejaculatory function and bother due to ejaculatory function both showed sustained improvement as measured with the MSHQ-EjD. These effects were shown to be durable to 3 years ($P<.001$).[9]

The erectile function effects of BPH procedures have long been debated, with results varying from significant iatrogenic dysfunction to improvement after TURP.[1,25–29] McVary and colleagues[24] looked at PUL effects on erectile function by parsing the data into quartiles based on the baseline SHIM score. The data showed that men entering the study with moderate erectile dysfunction (ED) or normal function were unaffected by PUL, but men who originally had severe ED showed some improvement. As LUTS are an independent predictor of ED, it was hypothesized that erectile function improvement may be a reflection of improving LUTS or a regression to the mean without causing iatrogenic damage, such as neural ablation from errant heating. For both erectile and ejaculatory function, improvements were modest; the most important takeaway is that PUL does not seem to have a negative effect on sexual function.

Durability

The PUL procedure has been shown to offer sustained symptom relief, improved QoL, and increased urinary flow through at least 4 years (see **Fig. 9**, **Tables 2** and **3**). As is true of all LUTS therapies, some patients fail to respond and desire additional surgical intervention. TURP (unipolar and bipolar) and laser vaporization have been conducted on small cohorts of patients with UroLift implants. These procedures were conducted in routine fashion without complications due to the presence of the UroLift implants.[12,15] Additionally, there a some reports of radical prostatectomy years after UroLift implantation; these procedures were also conducted routinely with report of preservation of dissection planes.[30]

As is common with the development of any surgical technique, durability has improved with PUL over the years. In the safety and feasibility study before technique refinement, the 2-year retreatment rate was 13 of 64 enrolled patients (20%).[15] With advancements in surgical approach, the retreatment rate improved, with 1-year rates for the LIFT study (7 of 140 enrolled, 5%), crossover trial (1 of 53 enrolled, 2%), and BPH6 trial (3 of 44 enrolled, 7%) reflecting technique improvements.[12,13,19] The LIFT randomized study data are now available to 4 years. Surgical retreatment reported after UroLift procedure increased from 5.0% at 1 year to 10.7% at 3 years and 13.6% at 4 years of the 140 originally enrolled subjects.[9,12] This finding shows significantly greater durability than that reported for thermal ablation techniques, whereby 3-year surgical retreatment has been reported to range between 20% and 50%.[9] Unfortunately the definition of retreatment is not always clearly identified in the literature. It may include a different procedure or repeat of the same surgery, and/or treatment with medication. Reported retreatment rates as a consequence are not immediately comparable.

SUMMARY

The experience with the PUL procedure includes 10 years of clinical experience. The largest randomized study data demonstrate durability to at least 4 years. The treatment has been adopted by the regulatory bodies and insurance systems of multiple countries, including the United States.

The overarching goal of a minimally invasive therapy is to offer a therapeutic response superior to medical therapy while avoiding the complications of surgery. Additionally, minimally invasive solutions target an improvement in the overall patient experience and quality of care, from a lower risk site of service (office or surgery center) to a more rapid recovery and relief from bothersome symptoms. Clinical data demonstrate that PUL can be reliably performed under local anesthesia in the office setting. It typically results in rapid recovery without the need for postoperative urinary catheterization. Symptomatic and urinary flow improvements are both greater than medical therapy options but less than standard surgery. The complications of surgery, including iatrogenic sexual dysfunction, seem to be avoided with PUL. PUL's rate of recovery is superior, and patient satisfaction increases more quickly after PUL compared with TURP. A shortfall of many minimally invasive options is a lack of durability such that patients either require frequent retreatment or move on to standard surgery.

Adverse effects of PUL are typically mild to moderate and transient in nature. Encrustation of implant components can be avoided with proper placement of the device within the prostatic fossa. Removal of misplaced implants should be conducted during the index procedure using standard endoscopic retrieval tools. Implantation does not adversely affect subsequent transurethral procedures or other procedures involving the prostate. Sexual function after PUL is preserved, with no evidence of iatrogenic erectile or ejaculatory dysfunction reported in the clinical studies.

In summary, the level of evidence supporting PUL is high. The benefits of the treatment seem to be that PUL is local anesthesia compatible and offers a uniquely rapid response while preserving sexual function. Although LUTS and flow improvements are expected to be greater with standard surgery, the risk of complications, including sexual dysfunction, may not be acceptable to patients with BPH. It would seem that there is a significant population of men with BPH for whom PUL is a viable choice.

REFERENCES

1. Roehrborn C, McConnell J, Barry M, et al. American Urological Association guideline: management of benign prostatic hyperplasia (BPH). Linthicum (MD): American Urological Association Education and Research Inc; 2003.
2. Verhamme K, Dieleman J, Bleumink G, et al. Treatment strategies, patterns of drug use and treatment discontinuation in men with LUTS suggestive of benign prostatic hyperplasia: the triumph project. Eur Urol 2003;44:539–45.
3. Reich O, Gratzke C, Bachmann A, et al. Morbidity, mortality and early outcome of transurethral resection of the prostate: a prospective multicenter evaluation of 10,654 patients. J Urol 2008;180:246–9.
4. Bachmann A, Tubaro A, Barber N, et al. A European multicenter randomized noninferiority trial comparing 180 W Greenlight-XPS laser vaporization and transurethral resection of the prostate for the treatment of benign obstruction: 12-month results of the GOLIATH study. J Urol 2015;193:1–9.
5. Miano R, De Nunzio C, Asimakopoulos AD, et al. Treatment options for benign prostatic hyperplasia in older men. Med Sci Monit 2008;14(7): RA94–102.
6. Summary of Safety and Effectiveness, Prostalund CoreTherm Microwave Therapy System, PreMarket Approval (PMA) Number P010055.
7. Norby B, Nielsen HV, Frimodt-moller PC. Transurethral interstitial laser coagulation of the prostate and transurethral microwave thermotherapy vs transurethral resection or incision of the prostate: results of a randomized, controlled study in patients with symptomatic benign prostatic hyperplasia. BJU Int 2002;90:853–62.
8. Ahmed M, Bell T, Lawrence WT, et al. Transurethral microwave thermotherapy (Prostatron@version 2.5) compared with transurethral resection of the prostate for the treatment of benign prostatic hyperplasia: a randomized, controlled, parallel study. Br J Urol 1997;79:181–5.
9. Roehrborn C, Rukstalis D, Barkin J, et al. Three year results of the prostatic urethral L.I.F.T. study. Can J Urol 2015;22(3):7772–82.
10. Yu X, Elliott SP, Wilt TJ, et al. Practice patterns in benign prostatic hyperplasia surgical therapy: the dramatic increase in minimally invasive technologies. J Urol 2008;180:241.
11. Medicare data calculated from the Medicare Physician/Supplier Procedure Summary Master File, 2004-2007.
12. Roehrborn C, Gange S, Shore N, et al. Multi-center randomized controlled blinded study of the prostatic urethral lift for the treatment of LUTS associated with prostate enlargement due to BPH: the LIFT study. J Urol 2013;190(6):2161–7.
13. Sonksen J, Barber NH, Speakman M, et al. Prospective, randomized, multinational study of prostatic urethral life versus transurethral resection of the prostate: 12-month results from the BPH6 study. Eur Urol 2015;68(4):643–52.
14. Woo HH, Chin PT, McNicholas TA, et al. Safety and feasibility of the prostatic urethral lift: a novel, minimally invasive treatment for lower urinary tract symptoms (LUTS) secondary to benign prostatic hyperplasia (BPH). BJU Int 2011;108:82.
15. Chin PT, Boiton DM, Jack G, et al. Prostatic urethral lift: two-year results after treatment for lower urinary symptoms secondary to benign prostatic hyperplasia. Urology 2012;79:5.
16. Shore N, Freedman S, Gange S, et al. Prospective multi-center study elucidating patient experience after prostatic urethral lift. Can J Urol 2014;21: 7094–101.
17. McNicholas T, Woo H, Chin P, et al. Minimally invasive prostatic urethral lift: surgical technique and multinational study. Eur Urol 2013;64:292–9.
18. Mogensen K, Jacobsen J. The load on family and primary healthcare in the first six weeks after transurethral resection of the prostate. Scand J Urol Nephrol 2008;42:132–6.
19. Cantwell AL, Bogache WK, Richardson SF, et al. Multicentre prospective crossover study of the 'prostatic urethral lift' for the treatment of lower urinary tract symptoms secondary to benign prostatic hyperplasia. BJU Int 2014;113(4):615–22.
20. Wasson J, Reda D, Bruskewitz R, et al. A comparison of transurethral surgery with watchful waiting for moderate symptoms of benign prostatic hyperplasia. N Engl J Med 1995;332: 75–9.
21. Glass J, Bdesha A, Witherow R. Microwave thermotherapy: a long-term follow-up of 67 patients from a single centre. Br J Urol 1998;81:377–82.
22. Lau K, Li M, Foo K. Long-term follow-up of transurethral microwave thermotherapy. Urology 1998;52: 829–33.
23. Hill B, Belville W, Bruskewitz R, et al. Transurethral needle ablation versus transurethral resection of the prostate for the treatment of symptomatic benign prostatic hyperplasia: 5-year results of a prospective, randomized, multicenter clinical trial. J Urol 2004;171:2336–40.

24. McVary K, Gange S, Shore N, et al. Treatment of LUTS secondary to BPH while preserving sexual function: randomized controlled study of prostatic urethral lift. J Sex Med 2014;11:279–87.

25. Gravas S, Bachmann A, Reich O, et al. Critical review of lasers in benign prostatic hyperplasia (BPH). BJU Int 2011;107:1030–43.

26. Spailviero M, Strom KH, Gu X, et al. Does greenlight HPS laser photoselective vaporization prostatectomy affect sexual function? J Endourol 2010;24: 2051–7.

27. Frieben RW, Lin HC, Hinh PP, et al. The impact of minimally invasive surgeries for the treatment of symptomatic benign prostatic hyperplasia on male sexual function; a systematic review. Asian J Androl 2010;12:500–8.

28. Gupta N, Sivaramakrisna, Kumar R, et al. Comparison of standard transurethral resection, transurethral vapour resection and holmium laser enucleation of the prostate for managing benign prostatic hyperplasia >40 g. BJU Int 2006;97:85–9.

29. Montorsi F, Moncada I. Safety and tolerability of treatment for BPH. Eur Urol 2006;5:989–1024.

30. Roehrborn C, Gange S, Shore N, et al. Durability of the prostatic urethral lift: 2-year results of the L.I.F.T. study. Urol Pract 2015;2:1–7.

Convective Water Vapor Energy for Lower Urinary Tract Symptoms/Benign Prostatic Hyperplasia

Kenneth Jackson DeLay, MD[a], Kevin T. McVary, MD[b],*

KEYWORDS

- Benign prostatic hyperplasia • Bladder outlet obstruction • Lower urinary tract symptoms
- Convective water vapor energy

KEY POINTS

- Benign prostatic hyperplasia (BPH) is a histologic diagnosis that refers to the proliferation of smooth muscle and epithelial cells within the transition zone of the prostate.
- Half of men over the age of 40 develop histologic BPH. About half of men with BPH develop an enlarged prostate gland, called benign prostatic enlargement (BPE); among these, about half develop some degree of bladder outlet obstruction.
- Bladder outlet obstruction and/or changes in smooth muscle tone and resistance that can accompany BPH may result in lower urinary tract symptoms (LUTS).
- LUTS include storage disturbances (such as daytime urinary urgency, frequency, and nocturia) and/ or voiding disturbances (such as urinary hesitancy, weak urinary stream, straining to void, and prolonged voiding).
- Treatment requires either medical or surgical intervention. Efforts to use minimally invasive treatments for BPH have included transurethral microwave therapy, transurethral needle ablation, and the use of the prostatic urethral lift.
- Recent publication of 1-year data shows convective water vapor as a promising improvement in both the subjective symptoms and the objective findings associated with symptomatic BPH while having negligible negative impact on erectile and ejaculatory function.

INTRODUCTION

Benign prostatic hyperplasia (BPH) is a frequently encountered chronic urologic condition that is associated with the development of lower urinary tract symptoms (LUTS) and impacts quality of life (QOL).[1] BPH prevalence increases with age and often requires either medical or surgical treatment and is associated with high costs in men older than 50 years of age.[2] Per the American Urological Association guidelines, men with moderate and severe BPH should be offered therapy.[3] Although transurethral resection of the prostate (TURP) is used less commonly in contemporary practice, it remains the gold standard for BPH refractory to medical management. Bipolar TURP is associated with less intraoperative adverse events than monopolar TURP. Unfortunately, many of the more efficacious surgical therapies for BPH are associated with a significant risk of ejaculatory dysfunction (EjD) and lesser risk of erectile dysfunction (ED). In particular, TURP causes EjD in approximately 65% of men and ED in less than 10%.[4,5]

[a] Department of Urology, Tulane University Health Sciences Center, New Orleans, LA, USA; [b] Division of Urology, Southern Illinois University School of Medicine, 301 North 8th Street, St John's Pavilion, PO Box 19665, Springfield, IL 62794, USA
* Corresponding author.
E-mail address: kmcvary@siumed.edu

Urol Clin N Am 43 (2016) 371–375
http://dx.doi.org/10.1016/j.ucl.2016.04.005
0094-0143/16/$ – see front matter © 2016 Elsevier Inc. All rights reserved.

Efforts to use minimally invasive treatments for BPH have included transurethral microwave therapy (TUMT), transurethral needle ablation (TUNA), and use of the prostatic urethral lift, among many other options.[6] TUMT and TUNA require a high temperature gradient to facilitate adequate temperature delivery (convection) to the prostatic adenoma to induce necrosis.[1] Both of these therapies are associated with limited durability. The Rezum System (NxThera, Inc, Maple Grove, MN, USA) uses convection to deliver energy to the prostate and induce necrosis and requires no thermal gradient. Water vapor disperses into the prostatic tissue. Recent publication of 1-year data shows a promising improvement in both the subjective symptoms and the objective findings associated with symptomatic BPH while having negligible negative impact on ED/EjD.[7]

REZUM SYSTEM

Thermal treatment using the Rezum system involves a radiofrequency energy source within the handle to generate water vapor that intercalates with prostatic tissue. Conduction is the transfer of heat from an area of higher temperature to lower temperature. TUMT and TUNA energy transfer is done via conductive transfer, which requires a higher energy gradient. Rezum uses convection, which is the movement of a heated gas or liquid within a space.

With the patient in lithotomy position, treatment is administered via a standard transurethral approach with rigid cystoscopy. Patients treated on trial had the procedure performed with the aid of oral medications or under intravenous sedation. Under direct visualization, a polyether ether ketone (PEEK) needle is used to deliver the vapor with 9-second injections and allows for targeted treatment (**Fig. 1**). The needle achieves a depth of 10 mm and circumferentially delivers the vapor. In the initial safety study, each lateral lobe received a mean of 4.6 injections. Twenty-two percent required treatment of their median lobe with a mean of 1.8 injections. The vapor enters the cellular interstices of the prostatic adenoma. The tissue treated with the vapor reaches 70°C to 80°C, which causes immediate cell death. Injections commence 1 cm from the bladder neck at the 3 o'clock and 9 o'clock positions and are spaced in 0.5- to 1.0-cm intervals.[8] Clearly, the number of injections required depends on prostate volume and anatomical configuration.

EFFECTS ON PROSTATIC ADENOMA

To assess the impact of Rezum on prostatic tissue, a safety study was performed in which both

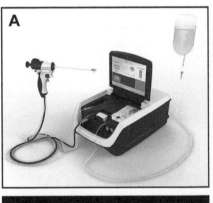
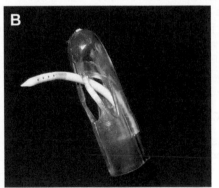
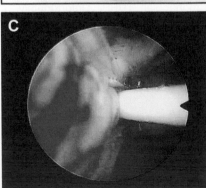
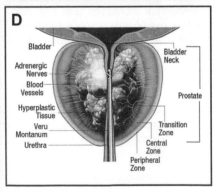

Fig. 1. (A) Rezum system. (B D) PEEK needle. (*Courtesy of* NxThera, Inc, Maple Grove, MN; with permission.)

histologic analysis and MRI were performed after Rezum therapy. Seven patients who were scheduled for simple prostatectomy underwent vapor therapy immediately before the procedure. Median prostatic volume was 39.8 cm³. Fresh examination of the prostatic tissue was performed after staining with triphenyl-tetrazolium chloride (TTC), which demarcates viable tissue from that which has been rendered nonviable (**Fig. 2**). No thermal damage was seen in the extraprostatic tissues of patients in this cohort. Lesions produced by Rezum therapy were identified with each lesion averaging 1.8 cm × 1.89 cm. On hematoxylin-eosin staining, there were sharp demarcations between viable and nonviable tissue with thrombosed vasculature in the nonviable tissue. In this study, the mean number of injections per lateral lobe was 2.3 (range 1–4).[9]

A second cohort of patients in this study underwent prostatic MRI 1 week after Rezum therapy. Necrotic lesions had coalesced at the time of imaging. The defects were localized to the transition zone (**Fig. 3**). The mean defect per lateral lobe was 9.6 cm³ with the largest defect being 35.1 cm³. The urethra remained preserved on imaging.[8]

A second imaging study by Mynderse and colleagues[10] performed gadolinium-enhanced MRI 1 week, 1 month, 3 months, and 6 months after Rezum therapy. The 44 patients from this study were treated in the Dominican Republic, the Czech Republic, or Sweden. Here, the mean number of injections per lateral lobe was 2.0. Imaging at 6 months showed a 28.9% and 38.0% reduction in the volume of the transition zone and whole prostate, respectively. At the 6-month mark, this reduction had progressed further to 95.1%. Based on volume calculations in patients who only received one injection per lobe, it appears that each injection causes a 1.7-cm³ lesion volume. In this study, the urethra was preserved in all patients, but 3 patients did show evidence of energy delivered outside of the prostate. All defects were at least 1.54 cm away from the rectal wall. This study did demonstrate a bounce in prostate-specific antigen (PSA) levels, which returned to baseline by 3 months.[10]

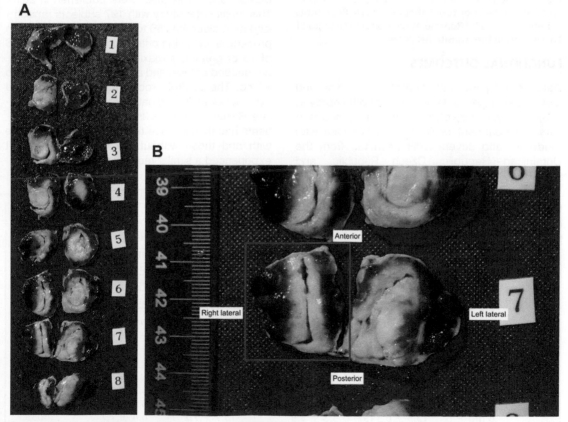

Fig. 2. Note that viable tissue takes up TTC. The transition zone shows no staining consistent with the tissue having been rendered necrotic.

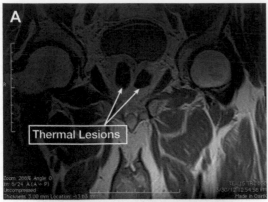

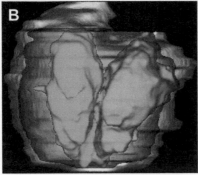

Fig. 3. Hypointense lesions within the prostate represent areas of necrotic tissue after Rezum. (*A*) Represents 2 thermal lesions (*B*) Represents reconstructed images of two lesions in the transitional zone.

FUNCTIONAL OUTCOMES

Data from a pilot study published by Dixon and colleagues[8] in 2015 demonstrated both improved subjective and objective parameters associated with the treatment of BPH. Sixty-five men with moderate and severe BPH (recruited from the Dominican Republic, Czech Republic, and

Sweden) were treated with Rezum as described earlier. Data regarding urinary symptoms as measured by the International Prostate Symptom Score (IPSS), peak urinary flow (Qmax), QOL, post void residual (PVR), erection quality as measured by the International Index of Erectile Function (IIEF), and PSA were collected. Data were collected at 1 week, 1, 3, 6 and 12 months after treatment. Subjects were unblinded at 6 months. IPSS improvement was noted at 1 month and maintained through 12 months with a 56% reduction overall. Qmax improvement was also noted at 1 month and persisted through the following period. It was increased by a mean of 87% over baseline at 12 months. Improvement in QOL scores were noted at all follow-up intervals. PVR reduction was present from 1 to 12 months. Improved IIEF scores were noted at 3, 6, and 12 months. Catheter duration was a mean of 5.6, although this was at physician discretion and could likely have been shortened. There was a 680% increase in PSA at 1 week of follow-up; however, this returned to baseline by 3 months. Urinary retention, dysuria, and urgency were the most commonly reported adverse events.[8]

The results of a randomized controlled trial by McVary and colleagues[7] were published in 2015. This multicenter study with 197 subjects randomized men older than 50 to either Rezum or a sham procedure. Inclusion criteria consisted of an IPSS of 13 or greater, a maximum flow rate of 15 mL per second or less, and a prostate size from 30 to 80 cc. The control procedure consisted of rigid cystoscopy in draped patients with noises to simulate Rezum treatment. In this trial, 31.1% of patients had median lobe tissue treated. Both those with and those without median lobe treatment experienced a similar reduction in IPSS (**Table 1**).

Table 1
Median lobe analysis

Measure	Time Point	Treatment No Median Lobe (N = 106) Mean ± Std (N)	Change Mean ± Std (N)	Treatment Median Lobe Treated (N = 30) Mean ± Std (N)	Change Mean ± Std (N)	P Value
IPSS	Baseline	21.9 ± 5.0 (106)	NA	22.4 ± 4.0 (30)	NA	NA
	3 mo	10.8 ± 6.9 (104)	−11.0 ± 7.7 (104)	9.9 ± 4.6 (30)	−12.5 ± 7.0 (30)	.3297
	6 mo	9.5 ± 6.1 (100)	−12.4 ± 7.5 (100)	10.8 ± 6.2 (29)	−11.5 ± 7.9 (29)	.5499
	12 mo	10.4 ± 6.8 (40)	−11.8 ± 6.5 (40)	9.0 ± 4.4 (3)	−9.7 ± 6.0 (3)	.5963
Qmax	Baseline	10.1 ± 2.3 (106)	NA	9.3 ± 2.0 (30)	NA	NA
	4 wk	13.3 ± 5.3 (104)	3.2 ± 5.0 (104)	12.5 ± 6.1 (29)	3.2 ± 5.9 (29)	.9861
	3 mo	16.0 ± 7.2 (104)	6.0 ± 6.9 (104)	16.3 ± 7.8 (29)	6.9 ± 7.8 (29)	.5206
	6 mo	15.3 ± 6.3 (97)	5.3 ± 5.9	15.7 ± 7.2	6.4 ± 7.7	.4033

Abbreviation: NA, not applicable.

Pain scores, as recorded by visual analogue score (VAS), did increase to a greater extent in those treated with Rezum versus control. Most patients received only oral sedation, although others did receive either a prostatic block or conscious intravenous sedation as well. Of the treated subjects, 90.4% were catheterized after the procedure for a mean of 3.4 days. Only 19.7% in the control group were catheterized, and the duration was shorter (mean of 0.9 days).

The primary endpoint of the trial was reduction in IPSS. At 3 months, 74% of subjects in the treatment group had an 8-point or greater reduction in IPSS versus 31% in the control group. This benefit was maintained at 12 months. Those with both moderate and severe LUTS experienced a benefit with Rezum. Twenty-two percent of patients had median lobe tissue treated. Both those with and those without median lobe treatment experienced a reduction in IPSS. Statistically significant improvement in Qmax and QOL scores was present from 3 to 12 months. Only 2 subjects in the treatment arm had serious adverse events (de novo urinary retention and persistent nausea/vomiting).[1]

IMPACT ON SEXUAL FUNCTION

Data regarding sexual function from the multicenter randomized trial by McVary and colleagues[7] have been published.[1] IIEF and Male Sexual Health Questionnaire (MSHQ)-EjD data were collected prospectively. There were no de novo cases of ED. There was no difference in IIEF-EF and MSHQ-EjD scores between the treatment and control group at 3 months. In the treatment group, 31% reported decreased EjD bother at 12 months compared with baseline. The minimal clinically important difference (MCID) in erectile function is based on baseline IIEF scores. Using these criteria, 32% and 27% of treatment subjects experienced an MCID improvement at 3 and 12 months, respectively. In contrast to TURP, Rezum treatment does not appear to cause ED or worsening of EjD. In fact, there is reduced EjD bother and potential improvement in ED in those treated with Rezum.

SUMMARY

Rezum is a novel therapy using convection energy transfer to cause necrosis of prostatic adenoma using water vapor. It is associated with minimal adverse events and minimal pain and can be performed without general anesthesia. After ablation of the adenoma, there is a statistically significant improvement in IPSS, QOL, Qmax, and PVR that is durable to 1 year. Short-term data show no worsening of ED or EjD. This technology represents a promising alternative in the treatment of BPH.

REFERENCES

1. Hahn DW, Ozisik MN. Heat conduction fundamentals, in heat conduction. 3rd edition. Hoboken (NJ): John Wiley & Sons, Inc.; 2012.

2. Fenter TC, Naslund MJ, Shah MB, et al. The cost of treating the 10 most prevalent diseases in men 50 years of age or older. Am J Manag Care 2006; 12(Suppl 4):90.

3. Available at: https://www.auanet.org/common/pdf/education/clinical-guidance/Benign-Prostatic-Hyperplasia.pdf. Accessed May 11, 2016.

4. AUA Practice Guidelines Committee for the American Urological Association. AUA guideline on management of benign prostatic hyperplasia. Chapter 3: results of the treatment outcomes analyses. Linthincum (MD): American Urological Association; 2003.

5. Rassweiler J, Teber D, Kuntz R, et al. Complications of transurethral resection of the prostate (TURP)—incidence, management and prevention. Eur Urol 2006;50:969–80.

6. Gravas S, Bach T, Bachmann A, et al. Guidelines on the management of non-neurogenic male lower urinary tract symptoms (LUTS), Incl. benign prostatic obstruction (BPO). EAU guidelines. 2015. Available at: http://uroweb.org/wp-content/uploads/13-.

7. McVary KT, Gange SN, Gittelman MC, et al. Minimally invasive prostate convective water vapor energy (WAVE) ablation: a multicenter, randomized, controlled study for treatment of lower urinary tract symptoms secondary to benign prostatic hyperplasia. J Urol 2015. http://dx.doi.org/10.1016/j.juro.2015.10.181.

8. Dixon C, Cedano ER, Pacik D, et al. Efficacy and safety of Rezūm system water vapor treatment for lower urinary tract symptoms secondary to benign prostatic hyperplasia. Urology 2015;86(5):1042–7.

9. Dixon CM, Cedano ER, Mynderse LA, et al. Transurethral convection water vapor as a treatment for lower urinary tract symptomatology due to benign prostatic hyperplasia using the RezūmR system: evaluation of acute ablative capabilities in the human prostate. Res Rep Urol 2015;7:13.

10. Mynderse LA, Hanson D, Robb RA, et al. Rezūm system water vapor treatment for lower urinary tract symptoms/benign prostatic hyperplasia: validation of convective thermal energy transfer and characterization with magnetic resonance imaging and 3-dimensional renderings. Urology 2015;86:122.

Bipolar, Monopolar, Photovaporization of the Prostate, or Holmium Laser Enucleation of the Prostate
How to Choose What's Best?

Jean-Nicolas Cornu, MD, PhD, FEBU

KEYWORDS

- Benign prostatic obstruction • Laser • Resection • Enucleation • Vaporization

KEY POINTS

- Relief from benign prostatic obstruction is possible by enucleation, resection, or vaporization.
- Laser enucleation gives the best long term functional results, with low perioperative risk, but has a steep learning curve.
- GreenLight photovaporization is useful in patients at high risk of bleeding and with limited prostate volume.
- Bipolar resection is a safe alternative to monopolar resection with comparable outcomes and no limitation owing to prostate size.
- The field is evolving, with many of innovative techniques that may help to refine indications according to patients' profiles.

INTRODUCTION

Lower urinary tract symptoms owing to benign prostatic obstructions (BPO) are highly prevalent and a huge number of men undergo surgery for BPO relief each year.[1] Among available options, aside traditional monopolar transurethral resection of the prostate (M-TURP) and open prostatectomy, many surgical options have been validated and are available for use in current clinical practice.[2,3] Transurethral ablative therapies are based on 3 different approaches: resection, vaporization (eventually combined in vaporesection), or enucleation. Available tools include monopolar energy, bipolar energy, holmium laser, photovaporization of the prostate (PVP; GreenLight) laser, and other less studied energy sources (thulium lasers, diode laser, etc). To date, the following surgical techniques have been validated through level 1 evidence studies: M-TURP, bipolar TURP (B-TURP), transurethral bipolar enucleation (TUBE), holmium laser enucleation of the prostate (HoLEP), and GreenLight PVP, as well as thulium vaporesection and enucleation.[2–4]

The respective results of each technique in currently available randomized, controlled trials (RCTs), in terms of BPO relief and tissue removal, seems more related to the type of tissue ablation chosen. Indeed, enucleation is associated with a higher amount of prostatic tissue removed, greater decrease in prostate-specific antigen, more improved peak flow rate (Q_{max}), and greater

Conflicts of Interest: J.-N. Cornu has received honoraria/travel grants from Astellas, Pfizer, Coloplast, AMS, Mundipharma, BARD, GSK, BK Medical, Allergan, EDAP-TMS.
Department of Urology, Rouen University Hospital, University of Rouen, 1 Rue de Germont, Cedex 1, Rouen 76031, France
E-mail address: Jeannicolas.cornu@gmail.com

change in International Prostate Symptom Score (I-PSS); results of resection and PVP seem comparable.[2-6] However, long-term data and some head-to-head comparisons are still missing. Furthermore, these techniques offer different types and/or rates of immediate or late complications. Their respective indications rely on patients' characteristics (risk of bleeding, life expectancy, and associated conditions), patients' expectations (notably in sexually active patients), and expertise of the surgeons (habits, learning curve, availability of the devices).

This paper aims to provide the best up-to-date information on the 4 major surgical transurethral techniques available on the market, to help urologists in choosing between M-TURP, B-TURP/TUBE, GreenLight PVP, and HoLEP. A cost-effectiveness analysis was considered to be out of the scope of this paper.

MONOPOLAR TRANSURETHRAL RESECTION OF THE PROSTATE
Indications

M-TURP is considered as a standard procedure for BPO relief, and has now been used for more than 7 decades. One of its main assets is the large clinical experience available in the literature, because nearly all urologists do M-TURP on a daily basis. M-TURP has thus been used as the reference treatment arm in more than 200 comparative studies in the past 30 years. However, owing to the need of glycine continuous flow irrigation the procedure, it is usually recommended to use M-TURP for prostates of less than 80 mL.[5] Furthermore, several RCTs and metaanalyses have shown that M-TURP is associated with a higher risk of bleeding compared with laser surgery (either PVP or HoLEP).[2,7,8] It may explain that no RCT have compared M-TURP with laser procedures in patients under anticoagulation, therapy likely owing to ethical reasons. At present, M-TURP remains an option for BPO relief in patients with small prostates (when the risk of bleeding is minimal) or in patients with voiding difficulties in the context of known prostate cancer.

Functional Results

It has been shown by numerous studies that M-TURP is able to relieve BPO with a high success rate. The procedure is associated with a drop in the I-PSS of around 70%, a reduction of prostate volume of around 45%, an increase of Q_{max} of around 12 mL/s, and a reduction is postvoid residual volume (PVR) of around 76%.[2,9-11] Those results are durable with an overall estimated

recurrence of BPO in about 10% of cases in the long term.

Complications

Intraoperative complications are dominated by bleeding, with rates between 3% and 8.6%, depending on the type of patients studied and whether it is in current clinical practice or clinical trials.[2,9-13] The risk of bleeding is even greater under anticoagulation therapy. TUR syndrome may occur in as many as 1% to 2% of patients owing to dilutional hyponatremia and is characterized by mental confusion, nausea, vomiting, and visual disturbances. It has been reported to occur in as many as 1% and 2% of cases.[2,9]

Postoperative clot retention owing to bleeding occurs in 1% to 7% of patients reported in the literature.[9] This complication is influenced by technical difficulties, prostate size, venous injury, depth of resection, and irrigation quantity after the procedure. Obviously, patients under anticoagulation therapy are at greater risk. Postoperative acute urinary retention can occur in 3% to up to 9% of cases.[2,9-12] It may be transient or impossible after further trials of voiding without catheter. In these cases, reevaluation of the patient by endoscopy and urodynamics is mandatory because many other factors can explain the situation (detrusor impairment, insufficient tissue removal). Urinary tract infections (UTIs) are usually successfully managed by antibiotics[2,9,11] and occur in up to 20% of patients. Some authors have proposed that preoperative bacteriuria, duration of the procedure, postoperative stay duration, and postoperative invasive care were linked to an increased rate of UTIs. Further complications can occur but are not frequent, underreported, and not seen in small RCTs in the literature. Those include perforation of the bladder neck, injury of ureteral orifices, and bladder wall injury. Mortality of the procedure is estimated to be around 1 in 1000 in the largest case series.[10]

Long-term complications include mainly bladder neck contracture, urethral strictures, incontinence, and sexual dysfunction. Bladder neck contracture occurs rather after TRUP in small prostates around 3% in the literature ($\leq$10%), and are managed successfully by incisions.[2,9,11] Urethral strictures occur in 2% to 10% of cases in the literature,[2,9,11] and are probably influenced by the size of the scope, the technology used, as well as UTIs. Urethral stricture is usually managed by laser of cold knife incision. Incontinence after TURP is rather unusual, is mainly owing to sphincter injury, and occurs in up to 2% of cases.[2,9,11] Reoperation rates depend on follow-up duration. It ranges from 3% to 14% in the long term (probably around 10%).[2,9,11] Erection is probably not really impacted by the procedure. Retrograde ejaculation is common (around 50%).[2,9,11]

Learning Curve

Despite its high popularity, the learning curve of TURP has not been deeply investigated in the literature. M-TURP has a learning curve like every urologic procedure. Some authors found that 80 procedures were needed to get a plateau in the learning curve, when postoperative outcomes were analysed.[14] Some simulation models have been proposed[15] but not thoroughly investigated.

BIPOLAR PROCEDURES
Indications

Bipolar procedures have been proposed initially as a variant of TURP using electric energy but using a bipolar electrode, allowing power up to 400 W. Several devices have been marketed to date (Gyrus, ACMI, Olympus, Karl Storz). Thanks to saline irrigation, innovative design of the resection loops, resection (B-TURP), but also vaporization (TUVP) and enucleation (TUBE) are possible with bipolar devices.

Functional Results

B-TURP has been shown to provide similar results compared with M-TURP in all systematic reviews and metaanalyses. Level 1 evidence has shown that this procedure is associated with a decrease in the I-PSS of around 71%, a reduction of prostate volume of around 46%, an increase of Q_{max} of around 13 mL/s, and a reduction is PVR of around 82%. The limited evidence available about bipolar enucleation shows that the procedure removes more prostatic tissue and is probably more comparable with HoLEP, but more information from well-designed prospective studies are required. Long-term data are lacking for B-TURP and TUBE.

Complications

Intraoperative complications of B-TURP are minimal given the absence of TURP syndrome. Bleeding is the main concern, but the risk of transfusion is reduced by 50% compared with M-TURP. Hemoglobin loss is also significantly reduced, as well as clot retention. Other complication rates are similar than after M-TURP. Long-term complications are similar to TURP (urethral stenosis, bladder neck contracture, reoperation, and incontinence, which is very uncommon).

Sexual dysfunction is mostly owing to ejaculatory dysfunction (around 60% of cases).

Learning Curve

Very few data have been published about the B-TURP and TUBE learning curves.[16] One possible explanation for this is the absence of standardization of the technique, especially for the enucleation technique. Several groups reported different tools, various loops, energy settings, and occasionally morcellation (using a morcellator or the mushroom technique). B-TURP procedure is likely comparable with TURP, but the TUBE procedure is better described and standardized.

GREENLIGHT PHOTOVAPORIZATION OF THE PROSTATE
Indications

PVP has emerged in the last 10 years with 2 consecutive modifications of the device, that is now delivering a power up to 180W in a specially designed fiber with integrated cooling system. The intervention is made using a continuous flow resectoscope with saline irrigation. GreenLight laser (532 nm wavelength, quasicontinuous mode) is able to vaporize tissue and coagulate, so that no material is available for pathology. Prostate size is theoretically unlimited, but current level 1 evidence is only available for prostates of less than 100 mL. The main attribute of GreenLight laser is in its hemostasis properties. The targeted chromophore is hemoglobin, with a very high absorption coefficient.[17,18] Tissue penetration of the laser is 0.8 mm. The main indication for GreenLight laser today is rather small prostates in frail patients with a high risk of bleeding (anticoagulation therapy or antiplatelets) or limited life expectancy and many comorbidities (level 1 evidence European Association of Urology guidelines[4]). There is no clear reference for what to do with anticoagulation therapy in these cases (suspend, bridging, or continue). Furthermore, there are no data about PVP and the new oral anticoagulants.

Functional Results

Short-term results[5] have shown that PVP was noninferior to TURP for symptoms improvement and BPO relief, that had been anticipated by others before the release of the GOLIATH study. The procedure is associated with a decrease in the I-PSS of around 66%, a decrease of prostate volume of around 44%, an increase of Q_{max} of around 12 mL/s, and a decrease in PVR of around 84%.[2] Long-term results are urgently awaited. This issue remains crucial as some reports about now 5 years of follow-up with the first generation of lasers were associated with a high recurrence rate.

Complications

Intraoperative complications are not frequent during PVP. Bleeding is significantly reduced with a very low rate of transfusion (1 case in the 7 RCTs available to date[5,19–24]). Intervention duration has been shown to be longer than TURP, but the difference was not clinically relevant (<10 minutes). The rate of UTIs was comparable with TURP as well as the risk of postoperative AUR. However, catheterization duration was reduced by almost 1 day and hospitalization duration reduced by 2 days. PVP is thus usually considered as a technique associated with the lowest hospital stay duration.[2]

Delayed hematuria has been presented recently as a potential issue during the first postoperative month after PVP.[25] Postoperative irritative symptoms are comparable with TURP when using appropriate evaluation. The major issue in long term follow-up with PVP is the reoperation rate that has been shown to be a bit higher than after TURP when evaluating medium term outcomes with the 120 W model,[2] whereas 18% recurrence of adenoma has been shown after 5 years of follow-up with an 80 W device.[26] Ejaculatory dysfunction has been reported in fewer case than after other techniques.

Learning Curve

The learning curve of PVP has not been yet adequately described. Although PVP is considered a relatively simple technique to learn,[10] some authors have pointed out that appropriate training is necessary.[27] The same authors have detailed PVP learning curve, and have shown that performance may continue to improve until up to 120 procedures.[28] To our knowledge, no rigorous evaluation of a curriculum integration training modules on exercise on the PVP simulator has been conducted.

HOLMIUM ENUCLEATION OF THE PROSTATE
Indications

HoLEP is the gold standard of transurethral enucleation of the prostate. By removing most of the adenoma, enucleation provides the best results possible in terms of BPO relief and long-term efficacy. This goal is virtually achieved by every other enucleation technique provided that the good plane is considered during the surgical procedures. Morcellation allows removal of the prostate tissue off the bladder and makes it available for pathologic examination. HoLEP is

the treatment of choice for enucleation, no matter the size of the prostate[2,29,30] Owing to its favorable profile regarding hemostasis, HoLEP is also indicated in patients at high risk for bleeding, under anticoagulation therapy, and in frail patients.

Functional Results

HoLEP has been found to provide optimal BPO relief with better functional outcomes than TURP and comparable outcomes with open prostatectomy.[2] The procedure is associated with a decrease in the I-PSS of around 78%, a decrease in prostate volume of around 59%, an increase of Q_{max} of around 17 mL/s, and a decrease in PVR of around 85%.[2] Long-term reoperation rates for BPO recurrence are minimal.[31]

Complications

Intraoperative complications include technical failures, wrong plane, or injury of the urinary sphincter. The ability to complete the procedure in a reasonable time span (<90 minutes) is of course influenced by the learning curve. Operative time has been shown to be a big longer than open prostatectomy and TURP even in experienced hands.[32–34] Immediate complications rate is lower after HoLEP with virtually no transfusion, and less postoperative bleeding compared with TURP and open prostatectomy. Rates of postoperative urinary retention, recatheterization, and postoperative UTIs are, however, comparable with TURP when HoLEP is used for smaller prostates. However, catheterization time and duration of hospital stay are greatly reduced. Postoperative transient incontinence is not uncommon after HoLEP and occurs in 1.3% to up to 20% of cases.[35] Older age, greater prostate size, and longer operative time have been shown as potential predictive factors for transient urinary incontinence.[35,36] In most cases, more than 80% of patients recover complete continence after a few months, and definitive incontinence is rather uncommon in the absence of a technical mistake during the procedure. Although erection seems not impacted by enucleation, HoLEP has been shown to be associated with a very high rate of ejaculatory disorders (>70%).

Long-term complications such as urethral strictures have shown comparable rates.

Learning Curve

Despite the numerous advantages of HoLEP, the discussions surrounding this technique is often about the initial learning curve of this procedure. The learning curve for HoLEP has been studied in several reports, with variables methods of assessment.[37–44] Published studies to date looked at technical success (complete enucleation, complete morcellation without technical failure or conversion for the procedure), operative time, complications, and functional outcomes. The numbers of cases required to reach the first step of the learning curve has been shown to be at least 20, and even 50 according to some authors. Data about operative time are heterogeneous, but this parameter surely improves with time; it is mostly influenced by patient selection (prostate size) and mentorship program. Complication rate and immediate outcome do not seem to be impacted dramatically by the learning curve in the initial phase. However, transient incontinence seems to decrease with greater experience. Some authors also point out that functional outcomes and complication rates may take a very long time to plateau.

Like other techniques (TURP and PVP), a HoLEP simulator has been proposed and the face and construct and validity of the model has been published.[45] However, no consistent data have been released in the field of clinical practice regarding the potential impact of training exercise on learning curve and future clinical practice. Furthermore, mentorship programs have been proposed but still improperly evaluated in term of impact on the learning curve.

SYNTHESIS

The pros and cons of each technique detailed in this article are gathered in **Table 1**. Although nearly 100 comparative clinical trials have compared the available options, some caveats still exist in the literature. First, some techniques have not been compared directly with others. Furthermore, data have been displayed in particular populations where the choice of the technique seems to impact the outcome: patients at risk of bleeding

Table 1
Assets and complication rate of each technique

	M-TURP	B-TURP	PVP	HoLEP
Level 1 evidence	Yes	Yes	Yes	Yes
Long-term data	Yes >15 y	Yes 5 y	Few	Yes >5 y
Prostate volume limit (mL)	80	No	100[a]	No
Duration of stay (d)[b]	4	3	2	2.5
Energy used	Electric current	Electric current	Laser 532 nm, quasicontinuous	Laser 2140 nm, pulsed
Operative time	—	—	—	—
Pathologic material	Yes	Yes	No	Yes
Early complications (%)				
TURP syndrome	1–2	No	No	No
Transfusion	5	2	0.2	0.8
Clot retention	6.3	3	1	2
Immediate AUR	5.7	4	5	5
Urinary tract infection	4	4.2	6	8
Delayed complications (%)				
Ejaculation disorders	60	60	35	>70
Bladder neck contracture	3	4	3	3
Urethral stricture	5	4.5	5	2
Persistent incontinence	1	<1	1	2

Abbreviations: AUR, acute urinary retentions; B-TURP, bipolar transurethral resection of the prostate; HoLEP, holmium laser enucleation of the prostate; M-TURP, monopolar transurethral resection of the prostate; PVP, photovaporization of the prostate; TURP, transurethral resection of the prostate.
Data are driven from randomized controlled trials.
[a] Some data have been published in case series about GreenLight photovaporization of the prostate for prostates greater than 100 mL, but with short-term follow-up and outside well-designed comparative trials.
[b] Median values, drawn from data published in available randomized controlled trials.[2]
Data from Cornu JN, Ahyai S, Bachmann A, et al. A systematic review and meta-analysis of functional outcomes and complications following transurethral procedures for lower urinary tract symptoms resulting from benign prostatic obstruction: an update. Eur Urol 2015;67(6):1066–96.

(especially patients under anticoagulation therapy), elderly patients (frail patients with a short life expectancy), patients requiring minimal impact of surgery on sexual function, and big prostates (>120 mL).

At present, enucleation (especially HoLEP) has shown to be suitable for any prostate size, and is associated with favorable outcomes in patients at risk of bleeding. It should thus be considered as the treatment of choice for large prostates, especially when other factors make the patient at risk of postoperative complications. PVP is the recommended treatment for patients with a limited prostate size, and frail patients with short life expectancy at high risk for bleeding. B-TURP can be considered as an alternative to traditional M-TURP whenever M-TURP would have otherwise been indicated. Of course enucleation, is preferable with large prostates. These data have to be put in perspective with the development of new minimally invasive approaches, which may change indications for invasive treatments.

REFERENCES

1. Lukacs B, Cornu JN, Aout M, et al. Management of lower urinary tract symptoms related to benign prostatic hyperplasia in real-life practice in France: a comprehensive population study. Eur Urol 2013; 64(3):493–501.
2. Cornu JN, Ahyai S, Bachmann A, et al. A systematic review and meta-analysis of functional outcomes and complications following transurethral procedures for lower urinary tract symptoms resulting from benign prostatic obstruction: an update. Eur Urol 2015;67(6):1066–96.
3. Cornu JN. Functional outcomes and complications following transurethral procedures for benign prostatic obstruction relief. AUA Update Series, 2016, Lesson 32.
4. EAU Guidelines on Treatment of Non-neurogenic Male LUTS. Available at: http://uroweb.org/guideline/treatment-of-non-neurogenic-male-luts/. Accessed February 1, 2016.
5. Thomas JA, Tubaro A, Barber N, et al. A multicenter randomized noninferiority trial comparing greenlight-XPS laser vaporization of the prostate and transurethral resection of the prostate for the treatment of benign prostatic obstruction: two-yr outcomes of the GOLIATH Study. Eur Urol 2016;69(1):94–102.
6. Zhou Y, Xue B, Mohammad NA, et al. Greenlight high-performance system (HPS) 120-W laser vaporization versus transurethral resection of the prostate for the treatment of benign prostatic hyperplasia: a meta-analysis of the published results of randomized controlled trials. Lasers Med Sci 2016;31(3): 485–95.
7. Li S, Zeng XT, Ruan XL, et al. Holmium laser enucleation versus transurethral resection in patients with benign prostate hyperplasia: an updated systematic review with meta-analysis and trial sequential analysis. PLoS One 2014;9(7):e101615.
8. Mayer EK, Kroeze SG, Chopra S, et al. Examining the 'gold standard': a comparative critical analysis of three consecutive decades of monopolar transurethral resection of the prostate (TURP) outcomes. BJU Int 2012;110(11):1595–601.
9. Reich O, Gratzke C, Bachmann A, et al, Urology Section of the Bavarian Working Group for Quality Assurance. Morbidity, mortality and early outcome of transurethral resection of the prostate: a prospective multicenter evaluation of 10,654 patients. J Urol 2008;180(1):246–9.
10. Naspro R, Bachmann A, Gilling P, et al. A review of the recent evidence (2006-2008) for 532-nm photoselective laser vaporisation and holmium laser enucleation of the prostate. Eur Urol 2009;55(6): 1345–57.
11. Rassweiler J, Teber D, Kuntz R, et al. Complications of transurethral resection of the prostate (TURP)–incidence, management, and prevention. Eur Urol 2006;50(5):969–79.
12. Madersbacher S, Marberger M. Is transurethral resection of the prostate still justified? BJU Int 1999;83(3):227–37.
13. Lourenco T, Armstrong N, N'Dow J, et al. Systematic review and economic modelling of effectiveness and cost utility of surgical treatments for men with benign prostatic enlargement. Health Technol Assess 2008; 12(35):iii, ix-x, 1–146, 169–515.
14. Furuya S, Furuya R, Ogura H, et al. A study of 4,031 patients of transurethral resection of the prostate performed by one surgeon: learning curve, surgical results and postoperative complications. Hinyokika Kiyo 2006;52(8):609–14.
15. Källström R, Hjertberg H, Svanvik J. Construct validity of a full procedure, virtual reality, real-time, simulation model for training in transurethral resection of the prostate. J Endourol 2010;24(1):109–15.
16. Xiong W, Sun M, Ran Q, et al. Learning curve for bipolar transurethral enucleation and resection of the prostate in saline for symptomatic benign prostatic hyperplasia: experience in the first 100 consecutive patients. Urol Int 2013;90(1):68–74.
17. Szlauer R, Götschl R, Razmaria A, et al. Endoscopic vaporesection of the prostate using the continuous-wave 2-microm thulium laser: outcome and demonstration of the surgical technique. Eur Urol 2009; 55(2):368–75.
18. Bach T, Muschter R, Sroka R, et al. Laser treatment of benign prostatic obstruction: basics and physical differences. Eur Urol 2012;61(2):317–25.
19. Al-Ansari A, Younes N, Sampige VP, et al. Green-Light HPS 120-W laser vaporization versus

transurethral resection of the prostate for treatment of benign prostatic hyperplasia: a randomized clinical trial with midterm follow-up. Eur Urol 2010; 58(3):349–55.

20. Lukacs B, Loeffler J, Bruyère F, et al, REVAPRO Study Group. Photoselective vaporization of the prostate with GreenLight 120-W laser compared with monopolar transurethral resection of the prostate: a multicenter randomized controlled trial. Eur Urol 2012;61(6):1165–73.

21. Capitán C, Blázquez C, Martin MD, et al. 120-W laser vaporization versus transurethral resection of the prostate for the treatment of lower urinary tract symptoms due to benign prostatic hyperplasia: a randomized clinical trial with 2-year follow-up. Eur Urol 2011;60(4):734–9.

22. Kumar A, Vasudeva P, Kumar N, et al. A prospective randomized comparative study of monopolar and bipolar transurethral resection of the prostate and photoselective vaporization of the prostate in patients who present with benign prostatic obstruction: a single center experience. J Endourol 2013;27(10):1245–53.

23. Pereira-Correia JA, de Moraes Sousa KD, Santos JB, et al. GreenLight HPS™ 120-W laser vaporization vs transurethral resection of the prostate (<60 mL): a 2-year randomized double-blind prospective urodynamic investigation. BJU Int 2012;110(8):1184–9.

24. Xue B, Zang Y, Zhang Y, et al. GreenLight HPS 120-W laser vaporization versus transurethral resection of the prostate for treatment of benign prostatic hyperplasia: a prospective randomized trial. J Xray Sci Technol 2013;21(1):125–32.

25. Jackson RE, Casanova NF, Wallner LP, et al. Risk factors for delayed hematuria following photoselective vaporization of the prostate. J Urol 2013; 190(3):903–8.

26. Guo S, Müller G, Lehmann K, et al. The 80-W KTP GreenLight laser vaporization of the prostate versus transurethral resection of the prostate (TURP): adjusted analysis of 5-year results of a prospective non-randomized bi-center study. Lasers Med Sci 2015;30(3):1147–51.

27. Misrai V, Faron M, Elman B, et al. Greenlight photoselective vaporization for benign prostatic hyperplasia: analysis of the learning curve and contribution of transrectal ultrasound monitoring. Prog Urol 2013; 23(10):869–76.

28. Misraï V, Faron M, Guillotreau J, et al. Assessment of the learning curves for photoselective vaporization of the prostate using GreenLight™ 180-Watt-XPS laser therapy: defining the intra-operative parameters within a prospective cohort. World J Urol 2014;32(2):539–44.

29. Krambeck AE, Handa SE, Lingeman JE. Holmium laser enucleation of the prostate for prostates larger than 175 grams. J Endourol 2010;24(3):433–7.

30. Humphreys MR, Miller NL, Handa SE, et al. Holmium laser enucleation of the prostate–outcomes independent of prostate size? J Urol 2008;180(6): 2431–5.

31. Gilling PJ, Wilson LC, King CJ, et al. Long-term results of a randomized trial comparing holmium laser enucleation of the prostate and transurethral resection of the prostate: results at 7 years. BJU Int 2012;109(3):408–11.

32. Kuntz RM, Lehrich K, Ahyai SA. Holmium laser enucleation of the prostate versus open prostatectomy for prostates greater than 100 grams: 5-year follow-up results of a randomised clinical trial. Eur Urol 2008;53(1):160–6.

33. Naspro R, Suardi N, Salonia A, et al. Holmium laser enucleation of the prostate versus open prostatectomy for prostates >70 g: 24-month follow-up. Eur Urol 2006;50(3):563–8.

34. Salonia A, Suardi N, Naspro R, et al. Holmium laser enucleation versus open prostatectomy for benign prostatic hyperplasia: an inpatient cost analysis. Urology 2006;68(2):302–6.

35. Nam JK, Kim HW, Lee DH, et al. Risk factors for transient urinary incontinence after Holmium laser enucleation of the prostate. World J Mens Health 2015;33(2):88–94.

36. Elmansy HM, Kotb A, Elhilali MM. Is there a way to predict stress urinary incontinence after holmium laser enucleation of the prostate? J Urol 2011; 186(5):1977–81.

37. El-Hakim A, Elhilali MM. Holmium laser enucleation of the prostate can be taught: the first learning experience. BJU Int 2002;90:863–9.

38. Seki N, Mochida O, Kinukawa N, et al. Holmium laser enucleation for prostatic adenoma: analysis of learning curve over the course of 70 consecutive cases. J Urol 2003;170:1847–50.

39. Shah HN, Mahajan AP, Sodha HS, et al. Prospective evaluation of the learning curve for holmium laser enucleation of the prostate. J Urol 2007;177: 1468–74.

40. Elzayat EA, Elhilali MM. Holmium laser enucleation of the prostate (HoLEP): long-term results, reoperation rate, and possible impact of the learning curve. Eur Urol 2007;52:1465–71.

41. Bae J, Oh SJ, Paick JS. The learning curve for holmium laser enucleation of the prostate: a single-center experience. Korean J Urol 2010;51: 688–93.

42. Jeong CW, Oh JK, Cho MC, et al. Enucleation ratio efficacy might be a better predictor to assess learning curve of holmium laser enucleation of the prostate. Int Braz J Urol 2012;38:362–71.

43. Robert G, Cornu JN, Fourmarier M, et al. Multicenter prospective evaluation of the learning curve of the holmium laser enucleation of the prostate (HoLEP). BJU 2016. http://dx.doi.org/10.1111/bju.13124.

44. Brunckhorst O, Ahmed K, Nehikhare O, et al. Evaluation of the learning curve for holmium laser enucleation of the prostate using multiple outcome measures. Urology 2015;86(4):824–9.

45. Aydin A, Ahmed K, Brewin J, et al. Face and content validation of the prostatic hyperplasia model and holmium laser surgery simulator. J Surg Educ 2014;71:339–44.

Robotic-Assisted Simple Prostatectomy: An Overview

Marc Holden, MD, J. Kellogg Parsons, MD, MHS*

KEYWORDS

- Robotic surgery • Simple prostatectomy • Minimally invasive • Benign prostatic hyperplasia

KEY POINTS

- Simple prostatectomy performed by any approach declined in the last 15 years.
- In 2012, 5% of all simple prostatectomies were performed laparoscopically in the US.
- Few large series limited to robotic prostatectomies have been published, with limited data on retreatment rates.
- However, existing data suggest that robotic prostatectomy is associated with equivalent functional outcomes, a significant reduction in transfusion rates, decreased hospital length of stay, and no difference in hospital charges compare to the open approach.

INTRODUCTION

Despite widespread use of medical therapy, the global incidence and prevalence of benign prostatic hyperplasia (BPH) and lower urinary tract symptoms have increased in the past 2 decades. At least 6.5 million men in the Unites States and 1.1 billion men globally suffer from BPH.[1–4]

Factors likely driving these trends include an aging population and an increased prevalence of metabolic disorders such as diabetes, obesity, and the metabolic syndrome, all of which are associated with increased risks of BPH and lower urinary tract symptoms.[5–8] As a result, the incidence of BPH-associated adverse medical events has persisted and, in the case of urinary retention, possibly increased.[1,9,10]

Indications for BPH surgical therapy focus primarily on adverse medical events and include urinary retention, renal failure secondary to BPH, urinary infections, bladder calculi, hematuria, and failure of—or inability to tolerate—medications.[11–13] Thus, even in an era of BPH medical therapy, the need for BPH surgery persists.

In patients requiring surgery, EAU and AUA Guidelines recommend consideration of open simple prostatectomy (OSP) for the surgical treatment of patients with large volume (>80 mL) glands (www.EAU.org, www.AUA.org). Refined from transcapsular and transvesical techniques described by Freyer[14] and Millin,[15] OSP substantially improves International Prostate Symptoms Score, urinary flow rate, quality of life, and postvoid residual volumes.

However, OSP has also been associated with relatively high rates of perioperative transfusion, prolonged hospital duration of stay, reoperation, and urinary infections.[16–18] An analysis of the US Nationwide Inpatient Sample (NIS), for example, observed a transfusion prevalence of 21% among more than 6000 OSP procedures performed in the United States from 2008 to 2010.[19] In multiple single institution series, perioperative transfusion rates ranged from 3.3% to 36.8%, and perioperative mortality was as high as 2.1%. Other adverse events include clot retention, bladder neck contracture, wound infection, and myocardial infarction.[20]

Disclosures: None.

Division of Urologic Oncology, Department of Urology, Moores Cancer Center, University of California at San Diego, 3855 Health Sciences Drive, #0987, La Jolla, CA 92093-0987, USA

* Corresponding author.

E-mail address: k0parsons@ucsd.edu

urologic.theclinics.com

Robotic-assisted laparoscopic simple prostatectomy (RASP), first described by Sotelo and colleagues[21] in 2008, potentially improves perioperative outcomes for simple prostatectomy, and its use has been increasing. Two recent studies of the NIS examined trends in the use of simple prostatectomy.[19,22] From 1998 to 2012, there was an overall decrease in the number of simple prostatectomies performed, but a modest increase in the proportion of minimally invasive simple prostatectomies (up to 5% of all surgeries by 2012), although neither study could differentiate laparoscopic from robotic techniques.

Herein, we describe a technique for transvesical robotic-assisted prostatectomy and review published evidence of RASP outcomes.

SURGICAL TECHNIQUE

We describe a technique for suprapubic, transperitoneal RASP which emulates classic anatomic principles of suprapubic OSP.[21] Other investigators have described retropubic and preperitoneal approaches for RASP. There is no evidence in the literature to suggest that any one of these techniques is superior to the others.[23–25]

Preoperative Evaluation and Preparation

Judicious screening for prostate cancer should be considered per evidence-based recommendations (www.nccn.org). Although prostate adenocarcinoma has been reported in up to 10% of series of simple prostatectomy,[26] the clinical significance of this observation in the modern era is unclear.

Per evidence-based guidelines, transrectal ultrasonography, cystoscopy, and urodynamics may be considered, and may be helpful in establishing the need for simple prostatectomy. Documentation of prostate volume, intravesical protrusion of median lobe, diverticuli, and calculi may be noted. Standard considerations for the preoperative evaluation of a patient undergoing laparoscopy may be made. Bowel preparation is unnecessary.

Patient Setup

The patient is placed in the supine Trendelenburg position with the legs spread, identical to the positioning for a robotic-assisted radical prostatectomy, with a Foley catheter in the bladder and 5 or 6 ports placed across the lower abdomen: typically a camera port, three 8-mm arm ports, and a 12-mm assistant port (**Fig. 1**). The robot is docked in the standard fashion,

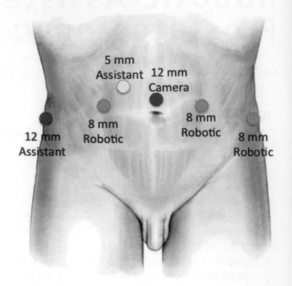

Fig. 1. Typical port placement. (*From* Patel M, Hemal A. Robot-assisted laparoscopic simple anatomic prostatectomy. Urol Clin North Am 2014;41:487; with permission.)

Prostate Exposure

In an initial approach identical to robotic-assisted radical prostatectomy, an incision is made in the anterior abdominal wall and the space of Retzius is accessed in the standard transperitoneal fashion. The medial and the median umbilical ligaments are transected and the bladder is released from the anterior abdominal wall. A transverse or vertical incision is made in the anterior bladder 2 to 3 cm proximal to the junction of the prostate and the bladder. The bladder lumen is entered, exposing the prostate adenoma.

Alternatively, the bladder is filled with normal saline to mark its boundaries and incised vertically on the posterior wall to enter the lumen. To provide fixed exposure of the bladder neck and prostate adenoma, the cystotomy incision is secured open with four 2-0 Vicryl sutures, 2 each placed at the anterior and posterior apices of the incision. The anterior and posterior sutures are secured in place to the anterior and lateral abdominal wall, respectively, with hemolock clips. The incision is lengthened as needed to afford additional exposure. Retraction sutures can be placed at the lateral margins of the cystotomy and affixed to the abdominal wall to facilitate exposure.[27]

Development of the Posterior Plane

To provide exposure of the posterior plane, the median lobe is placed on anterior traction by grasping it with the Prograsp forceps attached to the third arm of the robot. To minimize tissue tearing, we recommend placement of a 0 silk suture on a tapered needle through the adenoma in a figure-of-8 configuration, which then may be grasped with the forceps. The suture also facilitates dynamic repositioning of traction as the surgical plane develops circumferentially around the adenoma.

The bladder trigone and ureteral orifices are identified. A transverse, semicircular incision is made in the bladder mucosa along the posterior aspect of the adenoma corresponding with the posterior curve of the adenoma and the plane between the adenoma and capsule is entered. As the posterior plane between the adenoma and the peripheral zone is developed distally toward the prostatic apex, the bladder trigone and ureteral orifices drop posterior and cephalad.

Development of the Lateral and Anterior Planes

The mucosal incision is extended on the left and the right, first laterally, then anteriorly, such that the left and right extensions of the initial posterior incision are made to join anteriorly. Once the circumferential mucosal incision is completed, the plane between the adenoma and the peripheral zone is developed circumferentially in a distal fashion toward the prostate apex. Perforating vessels are cauterized with monopolar or bipolar energy as needed. The traction on the median lobe is repositioned as necessary to provide appropriate exposure; in general, continued cephalad traction will aid dissection.

Transection of the Urethra and Removal of the Adenoma

Once the adenoma is completely mobilized, the urethra is transected sharply at the apex under direct visualization, which allows urethral transection to occur well proximal to the external urinary sphincter. The adenoma is removed from the bladder and placed out of the operative field, for later extraction.

Advancement of the Bladder Neck Mucosa

The bladder neck mucosa is advanced to the distal urethral mucosa using 2 figure-of-eight 2-0 Vicryl sutures or as a continuous 3-0 monocryl V-lock suture.[28]

Bladder Closure

A 22-F or 24-F 3-way Foley catheter is placed under direct visual guidance into the lumen of the bladder. The bladder incision is then closed in multiple layers using a 3-0 Vicryl suture for the urothelium and 2-0 Vicryl for the detrusor muscle, both in a running fashion. If a transverse incision was made proximal to the bladder neck, the bladder incision is closed with a single full thickness 2-0 Monocryl suture in a running fashion. A Jackson-Pratt drain is placed. The Foley catheter is placed on traction, and consideration is given to initiating continuous bladder irrigation at a slow to moderate rate.

Postoperative Care

The catheter should be left to traction as needed for up to 2 hours after surgery, and continuous bladder irrigation should be used. Unless otherwise indicated clinically at an earlier time, hemoglobin and hematocrit are measured on the first postoperative day. If pain is well-controlled, laboratory test values are acceptable, and they are tolerating a diet, patients are discharged to home on postoperative day 1 with Foley catheter removal 1 week after surgery. A cystogram is not routinely obtained before catheter removal.

OUTCOMES

Robust analysis comparing outcomes between RASP and OSP is limited by a paucity of literature. There have been no randomized clinical trials (level 1 evidence). Also lacking are direct comparisons of RASP with HoLEP, the other surgical modality most often used for very large volume glands.

Still, at least 4 comparative cohort studies (level 2 evidence) comparing laparoscopic simple prostatectomy with OSP noted decreased blood loss, hospital duration of stay, catheter duration, and urinary infections for laparoscopic procedures.[29–31] Lucca and colleagues[32] recently published a metaanalysis of published series of minimally invasive simple prostatectomy that included RASP cases, identifying 27 studies published between 2004 and 2014 and reporting on perioperative and functional outcomes. In addition, a metaanalysis by Banapour and colleagues[33] identified 9 noncomparative case series (level 3 evidence) and represents the most comprehensive aggregation of perioperative and postoperative published RASP data to date.

Operative Time

Case series data consistently demonstrate longer operative times for RASP compared with published series of OSP, with mean operative times ranging from 90 to 228 minutes, and the majority being greater than 150 minutes (**Table 1**).

Table 1
Case series data for robotic simple prostatectomy

Series	Sotelo et al,[21] 2008	Yuh et al,[23] 2008	John et al,[34] 2009	Uffort et al,[41] 2010	Matei et al,[35] 2008	Sutherland et al,[36] 2011	Vora et al,[37] 2011	Matei et al,[38] 2012	Coelho et al,[39] 2012	Banapour et al,[33] 2014	Leslie et al,[27] 2014	Pokorny et al,[40] 2015	Autorino et al,[26] 2015
Patients (n)	7	3	13	15	15	9	13	35	6	16	25	67	487
Mean age (y)	64.7	76.7	70[a]	65.8	65.9	68	67.1	65.2	69	68.4	72.9	69	67
Mean operative time (min)	195	211	210[a]	128.8	180	183	179	186	90	228	214	97	145[a]
Mean operative blood loss (mL)	382	558	500[a]	140	50	206	219	121	208	197	143	200	200[a]
Transfusion prevalence, n (%)	1 (14.3)	1 (33)	0	0	0	0	0	0	0	0	1 (4)	1 (1.5)	5 (1)
Mean PSA (ng mL^{-1})	12.5	25	NR	5.2	NR	17.4	12.3	5.4	6.96	12.8	9.4	6.5	6.2[a]
Mean TRUS volume (mL)	77.7	323	NR	70.9	97.9	136.5	NR	106.6	157	141.8	149.6	129	110[a]
Mean resected prostate volume (g)	50.5	301	82	46.4	103.8	112	163.3	87	145	94.2	NR	84	75[a]
Mean length of stay (d)	1.3	1.3	6[a]	2.5	2.7	1.3	2.7	3.2	1	1.3	4.0	4	2[a]
Mean Foley duration (d)	7.5	NR	6[a]	4.6	7	13	8.8	7.4	4.8	8[a]	9	3	7[a]
Mean preoperative I-PSS	22	17.7	NR	23.9	NR	17.8	18.2	24[a]	19.8	22	23.9	25	23[a]
Mean postoperative I-PSS	7.25	NR	NR	8.13	NR	7.8	5.3	5[a]	1.1	7	3.6	3	7[a]

Abbreviations: I-PSS, International Prostate Symptom Score; PSA, prostate-specific antigen; TRUS, transrectal ultrasound.
[a] Median.

Operative Blood Loss and Transfusion

Compared with OSP, robot-assisted laparoscopic prostatectomy has been associated with substantially less blood loss and perioperative transfusion. The majority (85%) of robot-assisted laparoscopic prostatectomy series, and every series published after 2008, observed transfusion rates ranging from 0% to 5%; more than one-half (61%) observed a transfusion rate of 0%. The metaanalysis by Lucca and colleagues,[32] although not differentiating between laparoscopic and RASP outcomes, reported a transfusion rate of 6.4% for minimally invasive cases—much less than the 20% to 25% transfusion rates noted in OSP series.

Using the NIS, Parsons and colleagues[19] performed a direct comparison of 6027 OSP and 182 minimally invasive (laparoscopic plus RASP) cases and observed an adjusted transfusion prevalence 50% lower (odds ratio, 0.47; 95% CI, 0.18–1.26) for the minimally invasive approach. However, this difference did not attain significance ($P = .13$), likely in part because the analysis was study underpowered owing to the small number of minimally invasive cases.

Hospital Duration of Stay

Shorter duration of stay has been consistently noted in RASP, with most series reporting mean duration of stay ranging from 1 to 4 days (see **Table 1**). In the NIS series, the median duration of stay for RASP was 2 days less than OSP (2 vs 4 days), but the difference was not significant ($P = .19$), again, likely owing to an underpowered analysis.[19]

Complications

Given the variability in classification and reporting, comparison of complication rates is difficult, but there seem to be no substantial differences in complication rates between OSP and RASP (see **Table 1**).[19,26,32,33]

Duration of Catheterization

Although some comparative studies of laparoscopic to OSP noted decreased catheter duration for laparoscopic, there seem to be no substantial differences between catheter durations in published RASP and OSP series (see **Table 1**).

Functional Outcomes

Although long-term data and retreatment rates are not yet mature, perioperative and short-term functional data seem to demonstrate no substantial difference between OSP and the minimally invasive approaches, including RASP. Lucca and colleagues[32] reported an average aggregate improvement in the maximum urinary flow rate (Q_{max}) of 14.3 mL/s and International Prostate Symptoms Score improvement of 17.2 points for the minimally invasive approach, and identified 4 series directly comparing functional outcomes of open (n = 252 patients) and minimally invasive (n = 163 patients) approaches showing no differences in perioperative complication rates or changes in maximum urinary flow rate (Q_{max}) and International Prostate Symptoms Score after surgery.[19,33]

Cost Comparison

In an analysis of 35,171 prostatectomies in the NIS between 2002 and 2012, Pariser and colleagues[22] noted a significant difference in mean, inflation-adjusted hospital charges related to the presence of complications: $51,295 for patients with a complication versus $32,305 for patients without a complication. Without adjusting for complications, Parsons and colleagues noted no difference in mean hospital charges between OSP and minimally invasive simple prostatectomy.

SUMMARY

RASP is a safe and effective treatment for the management of symptomatic BPH in patients who are otherwise candidates for OSP. Cumulative level 3 evidence indicates low rates of perioperative transfusion, decreased duration of stay, and efficacy comparable with OSP. However, whereas initial level 2 evidence is possibly consistent with these observations, these data have not as yet demonstrated a statistically significant advantage for RASP for these outcomes. We therefore conclude that, although RASP has advanced beyond the experimental stage, definitive outcomes studies have yet to establish its benefits and costs relative to OSP and transurethral surgery.

REFERENCES

1. Wei JT, Calhoun E, Jacobsen SJ. Urologic diseases in America project: benign prostatic hyperplasia. J Urol 2008;179(Suppl 5):S75–80.
2. Irwin DE, Kopp ZS, Agatep B, et al. Worldwide prevalence estimates of lower urinary tract symptoms, overactive bladder, urinary incontinence and bladder outlet obstruction. BJU Int 2011;108: 1132–8.
3. Parsons JK, Bergstrom J, Silberstein J, et al. Prevalence and characteristics of lower urinary tract symptoms in men aged > or = 80 years. Urology 2008;72:318–21.

4. Parsons JK. Benign prostatic hyperplasia and male lower urinary tract symptoms: epidemiology and risk factors. Curr Bladder Dysfunct Rep 2010;5: 212–8.

5. Patel ND, Parsons JK. Epidemiology and etiology of benign prostatic hyperplasia and bladder outlet obstruction. Indian J Urol 2014;30:170–6.

6. Raheem O, Parsons JK. Associations of obesity, physical activity and diet with benign prostatic hyperplasia and lower urinary tract symptoms. Curr Opin Urol 2014;24:10–4.

7. McConnell JD, Roehrborn CG, Bautista OM, et al. The long-term effect of doxazosin, finasteride, and combination therapy on the clinical progression of benign prostatic hyperplasia. N Engl J Med 2003; 349(25):2387–98.

8. Kupelian V, Wei JT, O'Leary MP, et al. Prevalence of lower urinary tract symptoms and effect on quality of life in a racially and ethnically diverse random sample: The Boston Area Community Health (BACH) Survey. Arch Intern Med 2006;166:2381–7.

9. Stroup SP, Palazzi-Churas K, Kopp RP, et al. Trends in adverse events of benign prostatic hyperplasia (BPH) in the USA, 1998 to 2008. BJU Int 2012;109: 84–7.

10. Groves H, Chang D, Palazzi K, et al. The incidence of acute urinary retention secondary to BPH is increasing among California men. Prostate Cancer Prostatic Dis 2013;16:260–5.

11. McVary KT, Roehrborn CG, Avins AL, et al. Update on AUA guideline on the management of benign prostatic hyperplasia. J Urol 2011;185:1793–803.

12. de la Rosette JJ, Alivizatos G, Madersbacher S, et al. EAU guidelines on benign prostatic hyperplasia (BPH). Eur Urol 2001;40:256–63.

13. Parsons JK, Wilt TJ, Wang PY, et al. Progression of lower urinary tract symptoms in older men: a community based study. J Urol 2010;183:1915–20.

14. Freyer PJ. A new method of performing perineal prostatectomy. Br Med J 1900;2047:698–9.

15. Millin T. The surgery of prostatic obstructions. J Med Sci 1947;257:185–9.

16. Serretta V, Morgia G, Fondacaro L, et al. Open prostatectomy for benign prostatic enlargement in southern Europe in the late 1990s: a contemporary series of 1800 interventions. Urology 2002;60(4):623–7.

17. Gratzke C, Schlenker B, Seitz M, et al. Complications and early postoperative outcome after open prostatectomy in patients with benign prostatic enlargement: results of a prospective multicenter study. J Urol 2007;177(4):1419–22.

18. Suer E, Gokce I, Yaman O, et al. Open prostatectomy is still a valid option for large prostates: a high-volume, single-center experience. Urology 2008;72(1):90–4.

19. Parsons JK, Rangarajan S, Palazzi K, et al. A national, comparative analysis of perioperative outcomes of open and minimally invasive simple prostatectomy. J Endourol 2015;29:919–24.

20. Zargooshi J. Open prostatectomy for benign prostate hyperplasia: short-term outcome in 3000 consecutive patients. Prostate Cancer Prostatic Dis 2007;10:374–7.

21. Sotelo R, Clavijo R, Carmona O, et al. Robotic simple prostatectomy. J Urol 2008;179(2):513–5.

22. Pariser J, Pearce S, Patel S, et al. National trends of simple prostatectomy for benign prostatic hyperplasia with an analysis of risk factors for adverse perioperative outcomes. Urology 2015;86:721–6.

23. Yuh B, Laungani R, Perlmutter A, et al. Robot-assisted Millin's retropubic prostatectomy: case series. Can J Urol 2008;15(3):4101–5.

24. Stolzenburg J, Kallidonis P, Qazi H, et al. Extraperitoneal approach for robotic-assisted simple prostatectomy. Urology 2014;84:1099–105.

25. Patel M, Hemal A. Robot-assisted laparoscopic simple anatomic prostatectomy. Urol Clin North Am 2014;41:485–92.

26. Autorino R, Zarigar H, Mariano MB, et al. Perioperative outcomes of robotic and laparoscopic simple prostatectomy: a European-American multi-institutional analysis. Eur Urol 2015;68:86–94.

27. Leslie S, Abreu A, Chopra S, et al. Transvesical robotic simple prostatectomy: initial clinical experience. Eur Urol 2014;66:321–9.

28. Feretti M, Phillips J. Prostatectomy for benign prostate disease: open, laparoscopic, and robotic techniques. Can J Urol 2015;22(Suppl 1):60–6.

29. Rangarajan S, Palazzi K, Parsons J. Comparative outcomes of open and minimally invasive simple prostatectomy for symptomatic benign prostatic hyperplasia. J Urol 2014;191(4 Suppl):e789.

30. Baumert H, Ballaro A, Dugardin F, et al. Laparoscopic versus open simple prostatectomy: a comparative study. J Urol 2006;175(5):1691–4.

31. McCullough TC, Heldwein FL, Soon SJ, et al. Laparoscopic versus open simple prostatectomy: an evaluation of morbidity. J Endourol 2009;23(1):129–33.

32. Lucca IH, Shariat S, Hofbauer S, et al. Outcomes of minimally invasive simple prostatectomy for benign prostatic hyperplasia: a systematic review and meta-analysis. World J Urol 2015;33:563–70.

33. Banapour P, Patel N, Kane CJ, et al. Robotic-assisted simple prostatectomy: a systematic review and report of a single institution case series. Prostate Cancer Prostatic Dis 2014;17:1–5.

34. John H, Bucher C, Engel N, et al. Preperitoneal robotic prostate adenomectomy. Urology 2009;73(4): 811–5.

35. Matei DV, Spinelli MG, Nordio A, et al. Robotic simple prostatectomy. Eur Urol Suppl 2008;9:337.

36. Sutherland DE, Perez DS, Weeks DC. Robot-assisted simple prostatectomy for severe benign prostatic hyperplasia. J Endourol 2011;25(4):641–4.

37. Vora A, Mittal S, Hwang J, et al. Robot-assisted simple prostatectomy: multi-institutional outcomes for glands larger than 100 grams. J Endourol 2012;26(5):499–502.

38. Matei DV, Brescia A, Mazzoleni F, et al. Robot-assisted simple prostatectomy (RASP): does it make sense? BJU Int 2012;110(11 Pt C):E972–9.

39. Coelho RF, Chauhan S, Sivaraman A, et al. Modified technique of robotic-assisted simple prostatectomy: advantages of a vesico-urethral anastomosis. BJU Int 2012;109:426–33.

40. Pokorny M, Novara G, Guerts N, et al. Robot-assisted simple prostatectomy for treatment of lower urinary tract symptoms secondary to benign prostate enlargement: surgical technique and outcomes in a high-volume robotic centre. Eur Urol 2015;68(3): 451–7.

41. Uffort E, Jensen J. Robotic-assisted laparoscopic simple prostatectomy: an alternative minimal invasive approach for prostate adenoma. J Robotic Surg 2010;4:7–10.

Sexual Side Effects of Medical and Surgical Benign Prostatic Hyperplasia Treatments

Charles Welliver, MD[a,b,c,*], Ahmed Essa, MD[d,e,1]

KEYWORDS

- Benign prostatic hyperplasia • Lower urinary tract symptoms • Erectile dysfunction
- Ejaculatory dysfunction • Erectile function • Adverse events

KEY POINTS

- Sexual dysfunction in the cohort of men who seek treatment of lower urinary tract symptoms is common.
- Alpha blocker use frequently has effects on ejaculatory function with large difference in dysfunction rates based on medication selectivity.
- 5-alpha reductase inhibitor use may precipitate a variety of sexual adverse events with a complicated and layered pathophysiologic process.
- Surgical treatments frequently cause retrograde ejaculation with variation in incidence rates depending on the surgical treatment or technique.

INTRODUCTION

Lower urinary tract symptoms (LUTS) due to benign prostatic hyperplasia (BPH) are a common consultation for most practicing urologists. Although treatment rightly focuses on relief of urinary symptoms, the offered medical and surgical treatments frequently have unwanted effects that provoke sexual dysfunction in the forms of erectile dysfunction (ED) or ejaculatory dysfunction (EjD).

Despite the high prevalence of sexual dysfunction in the cohort of men who frequently require treatment of LUTS due to BPH,[1–6] sexual adverse events (AEs) of treatments are often inadequately assessed. These endpoints are often recorded by sporadic patient report and not by validated questionnaires. As a result, the true incidence and severity of ED or EjD with many of these treatments is only partially understood. Additionally, the effects of LUTS and increasing age on sexual dysfunction[1–6] makes interpretation of changes during the study period more challenging because new onset dysfunction may be related to treatment or natural age-related decline.

This article considers potential pathophysiologic causes of dysfunction with treatment of LUTS due to BPH and attempts to critically review the available data to assess sexually related AEs.

Disclosures: None (A. Essa). Honoraria, American Society of Andrology; consultant, Coloplast; investigator, Antares, NexMed, Auxilium, Sophiris, and PROCEPT BioRobotics; employee (brother), Bristol-Meyers Squib; compensated reviewer, Oakstone Publishing and BMJ Best Practice (C. Welliver).

[a] Division of Urology, Albany Medical College, 23 Hackett Boulevard, Albany, NY 12208, USA; [b] Division of Urology, Albany Stratton Veterans Affairs Medical Center, 113 Holland Ave, Albany, NY 12208, USA; [c] Division of Urology, Urological Institute of Northeastern New York, 23 Hackett Boulevard, Albany, NY 12208, USA; [d] Division of Urology, University of Al - Iraqi School of Medicine, Adhamyia, Haibetkhaoon, Street 22, District 308, Box office 7366, Baghdad, Iraq; [e] Department of Urology, Al-Numan Teaching Hospital, Adhamyia, Haibetkhaoon, Street 22, District 308, Box office 7366, Baghdad, Iraq
[1] Present address: Adhamyia, Haibetkhaoon, Street 22, District 308, Box office 7366, Baghdad, Iraq.
* Corresponding author. 23 Hackett Boulevard, Albany, NY 12208.
E-mail address: cwelliver@communitycare.com

Urol Clin N Am 43 (2016) 393–404
http://dx.doi.org/10.1016/j.ucl.2016.04.010
0094-0143/16/$ – see front matter Published by Elsevier Inc.

MEDICATIONS
Alpha Blockers

Alpha receptors are found throughout the human body, mostly as part of vascular smooth muscle and stromal tissue. In humans, there are 3 subtypes of alpha1 receptors: 1a, 1b, and 1d. Alpha1a receptor subtype comprises approximately 70% of prostatic alpha1 adrenergic receptors, with alpha1b generally found in systemic vasculature, although it has also been identified in the prostate.[7] Alpha1d receptors are found in the bladder and in the central nervous system where they may play role in central regulation of voiding.[8]

Alpha blockers (ABs) act by reversibly inhibiting receptor activation and are considered a first-line treatment of LUTS experienced secondary to BPH.[7] Having a firm understanding of receptor subtype and location helps explain the efficacy and side-effect profile of these commonly used drugs. The alpha1a subtype offers a promising target for lower urinary tract relaxation and obstruction relief, whereas action at 1b and 1d can produce systemic effects of vasodilation, including orthostatic hypotension and syncope. The different ABs are equally efficacious in reducing symptoms of BPH but differ in their side-effect profiles.[9,10]

AB medications can be roughly divided into selective and nonselective types. Third-generation ABs such as silodosin and tamsulosin have selective blockade, with silodosin acting specifically at alpha1a receptors and tamsulosin acting at both 1a and 1d. Nonselective ABs such as doxazosin and terazosin are not subtype specific and thus lead to more systemic side effects (headache, nasal congestion, syncope, orthostatic hypotension). These 2 medications produce fewer sexual AEs but must be titrated to mitigate their effects on orthostatic hypotension and syncope. The exception to this is alfuzosin, which is a nonselective AB that produces fewer first-dose systemic effects and does not need to be dose-titrated.[11]

The most common side effect of the ABs is EjD because alpha receptors are widely distributed in organs involved in the emission phase of ejaculation.[12] However, the previously held notion that EjD was due to relaxation of the bladder neck leading to retrograde ejaculation has been challenged. Although there are studies that still support the paradigm of retrograde movement of seminal fluid into the bladder with AB use, increasing evidence points towards anejaculation as the root cause.[13–15] Specifically, in vitro work on human vas deferens demonstrates alpha 1a receptor antagonism eliminates electrically induced contractions.[16,17]

As outlined in the American Urologic Association (AUA) guidelines for the treatment of BPH, sexual function is irregularly reported in most large AB studies.[9] A few studies to date have attempted to measure changes in sexual function beyond EjD in men taking ABs. See later discussion of nonselective and selective ABs as separate groups, and of studies comparing adverse effects between ABs.

Nonselective alpha blockers

The nonselective ABs include alfuzosin, terazosin, and doxazosin, and have a relatively low incidence of overall sexual dysfunction and EjD.[9,10]

One of the most rigorous examinations of the effects of a nonselective AB on various aspects of sexual function comes from the Medical Therapy of Prostatic Symptoms (MTOPS) trial data.[18] Five different domains of sexual function were examined using a validated questionnaire that was state of the art at that time. Doxasozin was the AB examined and minimal effects on sexual function were seen in subjects. In another trial looking at doxasozin in a randomized, controlled fashion, the incidence of EjD, decreased libido, and ED was not different between study and control groups with both reporting incidence of roughly 1%.[19]

In an uncontrolled study, 10 mg alfuzosin taken once daily for 1 year displayed improved ejaculatory function when compared with baseline measurements.[20] A study from the ALFORTI study group was a double-blind, controlled study that showed no significant difference in EjD, decreased libido, or ED between groups, adding further evidence to the low incidence of sexual side effects with nonselective ABs.[11] Another open-label study of 538 men taking 10 mg alfuzosin once daily over 2 years showed a small improvement in international index of erectile function (IIEF) score with no statistically significant difference in EjD or ED.[21]

Selective alpha blockers

More selective ABs, such as tamsulosin and silodosin, produce fewer systemic side effects but have a greater incidence of EjD. Multiple studies have demonstrated a subjective incidence of reported EjD between 4.5% to 11% with the 0.4 mg tamsulosin dose. However, there is no change in erectile function between treatment and placebo groups.[22–24] Slight improvements were noted in sexual desire, although differences in overall sexual satisfaction were not seen.[24]

There does seem to be a dose-EjD correlation in patients taking tamsulosin.[23] This was verified in a 2003 Cochrane review that found EjD in 18% of patients taking 0.8 mg dose tamsulosin, 6% in

0.4 mg group, and 0% in patients taking 0.2 mg dose.[25]

Theoretically, a drop in systemic blood pressure could induce ED, although studies examining changes in erectile function and ABs have not found an association. In a double-blind study over a 12 week period, tamsulosin was compared with placebo with a validated questionnaire. Although investigators found no difference in erectile function, they did note that men who were on tamsulosin had decreases in ejaculatory or orgasmic frequency and overall sexual satisfaction.[26]

Due to ultra-selectivity of silodosin, reported EjD rates have been among the highest seen for ABs. In a pooled analysis of 3 randomized placebo-controlled studies consisting of almost 1500 subjects, silodosin lead to 22% of subjects reporting EjD compared with only 0.9% of placebo patients.[27] A smaller, similar study in Japanese men found similar results with 22% of patients reporting EjD.[28]

Comparisons of alpha blocker medications

Although effects on urinary symptoms are often marginally different between ABs, the unintended effects with regard to both sexual dysfunction and systemic effects can be pronounced.

In a study conducted by Hellstrom and Sikka,[29] 48 healthy men were randomized to tamsulosin, alfuzosin, or placebo. In men taking 0.8 mg of tamsulosin, there was a 35% incidence of anejaculation, with 90% of men taking tamsulosin experiencing reduced semen volumes compared with only 21% of men on alfuzosin and 12.5% of men on placebo. No subjects in the alfuzosin or placebo groups suffered from anejaculation. A crossover study looking at tamsulosin and alfuzosin also found increased rates of EjD in patients treated with tamsulosin.[30]

Chapple and colleagues[31] reported EjD in a 3-arm study with 14.2% of subjects taking silodosin reporting symptoms compared with only 2.1% of those taking tamsulosin and 1.1% in the placebo group. In an attempt to gauge bother of the EjD, investigators looked at study discontinuation rates. Although statistical differences were not seen, more subjects discontinued the study in the silodosin group (5) than in the tamsulosin (1) or placebo (0) groups.

A meta-analysis by Gacci and colleagues[32] compared different ABs and their relative risk of producing EjD in men with LUTS. In comparison with placebo, increased risk was found with silodosin (odds ratio [OR] = 32.5) and tamsulosin (OR = 8.58). Doxazosin and terazosin did not have increased risk for EjD compared with placebo. Tamsulosin demonstrated less risk than silodosin in a direct comparison (OR = 0.09). Meta regression showed that EjD was associated with International Prostate Symptom Score (IPSS) and maximum urinary flow rate (Qmax) both before and after treatment, although analyses also showed that EjD was independently associated with improvement in IPSS and Qmax. **Table 1** summarizes the different AB study outcomes.

Table 1
Double-blind, randomized, placebo-controlled studies involving alpha blockers

Treatment	Subjects (Drug/Placebo)	ED (Drug/Placebo)	Decreased Libido (Drug/Placebo)	EjD (Drug/Placebo)
Alfuzosin 10 mg Qday[11]	143/154	0%/0.7%	0%/0.7%	0%/0%
Alfuzosin 2.5 mg TID[11]	150/154	0%/0.7%	0.7%/0.7%	0%/0%
Doxazosin[19]	275/269	5.8%/3.3%	3.6%/1.9%	3.6%/1.9%
Doxazosin[33]	3652/3489	3.56%/3.32%	1.56%/1.4%	1.1%/0.83%
Silodosin[28]	176/89	—	—	22%/0%
Silodosin[34,a]	466/457	—	—	28%/0.9%
Silodosin[27,a]	847/647	0.7%/0.3%	0.5%/0.2%	22%/0.9%
Tamsulosin 0.4 mg[23]	244/239	—	—	11%/<1%
Tamsulosin 0.8 mg[23]	248/239	—	—	18%/<1%
Tamsulosin[22]	381/193	0.8%/1.6%	1%/0%	4.5%/1%
Terazosin[35]	305/305	6%/5%	3%/1%	0.3%/1%

Open trial data is not included.
[a] These 2 studies have significant overlap in patient data.
Adapted from Welliver C, Butcher M, Potini Y, et al. Impact of alpha blocker, 5-alpha reductase inhibitors and combination therapy on sexual function. Curr Urol Rep 2014;15:441; with permission.

5-Alpha Reductase Inhibitors

Postulating a physiologic basis to sexual dysfunction

5-alpha reductase inhibitors (5ARIs) competitively inhibit the enzyme 5-alpha reductase (5AR), which is responsible for the conversion of testosterone to dihydrotestosterone (DHT). In the human body, there are 3 forms of the enzyme (types 1, 2, and 3), each concentrated in different organs and tissue types throughout the body. Although systemic AEs of 5ARI use are less often reported than those of AB, there is growing evidence of 5ARI action outside of the prostate.

The effects of 5ARIs primarily center on the augmentation of DHT levels but may have other indirect actions also. DHT is a potent androgen with important embryologic functions as well as functions in adults. Children born with 5AR deficiency demonstrate ambiguous genitalia and undermasculinization.[36] In adults, physiological levels of DHT promote prostate growth with a reduction in these levels specifically associated with involution of the epithelial component of the prostate.[37]

As more research emerges on the complex role androgens play in human physiology, a clearer picture of hormonal role in sexual function is beginning to unfold. Specifically, research has shown the androgens increase levels of nitric oxide (NO) synthase expression and DHT is more effective than testosterone at increasing expression, at least in rat models.[38] NO plays a critical role in increasing blood flow to the genitalia through its vasodilatory actions, allowing for proper erectile and ejaculatory function. One research team has postulated that lower levels of DHT, and the ensuing drop off in NO, lead to a deterioration in erectile function.[39] This theory has been corroborated by improvement in erectile quality in studies involving DHT supplementation in men.[40,41]

One explanation for the systemic, nonurologic effects of 5ARIs is the unintended influence of molecules called neurosteroids. 5ARIs not only prevent the conversion of testosterone to DHT but also inhibit the conversion of progesterone and deoxycorticosterone to their downstream important neurosteroid products. Psychological functions of neurosteroids are still being investigated but they have been postulated to have effects on mood, sleep, memory, anxiety, and sexual function.[42,43] Finasteride has demonstrated the ability to cross the blood-brain barrier and gain access to the central nervous system, where it could possibly affect the cognitive aspects of sexual drive and pleasure.

Further research is needed to elucidate this primarily associative relationship between 5ARI use and sexual dysfunction but it is a hypothesis and a not an unrealistic pathophysiology in the least. One specific example was a small study involving men treated with finasteride who were noted to have lower levels of 5AR neuroactive steroid levels in their cerebral spinal fluid. These products were associated with persistent sexual side effects and anxious or depressive symptoms.[44] It is hoped that further work will shed light on the specific mechanisms involved between 5ARI use and unintended systemic effects.

Study-specific outcomes

The FDA has approved 2 5ARIs, finasteride and dutasteride, for the treatment of BPH. Dutasteride inhibits both type 1 and 2 enzyme subtypes and finasteride is specific to type 2. Selective inhibition of type 2 receptor has been shown to reduce serum DHT by 70% to 80%, with decreases in intraprostatic DHT levels by 85%.[45,46] The dual inhibition of dutasteride is associated with both lower serum and intraprostatic DHT levels (90% and 95%) but also with a potentially more problematic side-effect profile.[46] Unlike ABs, 5ARIs are more clearly associated with sexual dysfunction beyond EjD, specifically decreased libido and erectile function, which seems to be most prominent after 1 year treatment with plateaus afterwards.[47,48]

Taking a general overview of large, placebo-controlled drug trials involving 5ARIs, multiple recurring themes are noted. Studies almost always use spontaneous, dichotomous (present or not present), subject-reported outcomes as opposed to validated questionnaires to assess change in sexual function. Most trial drug groups report a higher rate of symptoms in the active treatment group with regard to ED, EjD, and decreased libido. However, it should be noted that, although these differences are often statistically significant, usually there is less than a 3% difference in symptoms compared with placebo. Data from randomized, placebo controlled trials on 5ARIs can be found in **Table 2**.

Most changes in sexual function associated with 5ARI use are usually noted to peak at 1 year of treatment. Differences between placebo and treatment groups become less pronounced after that time and are often the same at study termination if trials last beyond 2 years. Although the exact mechanism for this is difficult to explain, it may be related to natural progression of sexual dysfunction that comes with age, as was observed in the placebo control groups in the previously mentioned MTOPS study.[18]

Table 2
Double-blind, randomized, placebo-controlled studies involving 5-alpha reductase inhibitors

Treatment	Subjects (Drug/Placebo)	ED (Drug/Placebo)	Decreased Libido (Drug/Placebo)	EjD (Drug/Placebo)
Dutasteride[49]	126/127	0%/1%	2%/0%	—
Dutasteride[50]	60/59	11%/3%	4%/2%	—
Dutasteride[51]	2167/2158	1.7%/1.2%	0.6%/0.3%	0.5%/0.1%
Dutasteride[52]	4105/4126	9%/5.7%	3.3%/1.6%	1.4%/0.2%
Dutasteride 1 y[47]	1510/1441	6%/3%	3.7%/1.9%	1.8%/0.7%
Dutasteride 2 y[47]	1510/1441	1.7%/1.2%	0.6%/0.3%	0.5%/0.1%
Finasteride[53]	1577/1591	6.6%/4.7%	4%/2.8%	2.1%/0.6%
Finasteride (1 mg)[54]	779/774	1.4%/0.9%	1.9%/1.3%	1%/0.4%
Finasteride (1 mg)[55]	133/123	0.75%/0%	1.5%/1.6%	0%/0.8%
Finasteride (1 mg)[56]	286/138	3.8%/0.7%	4.9%/4.4%	2.8%/0.7%
Finasteride[57]	1759/583	5.6%/2.2%	2.9%/1%	2.1%/0.5%
Finasteride[50]	55/59	11%/3%	13%/2%	—
Finasteride[58]	547/558	4.8%/1.8%	3.8%/2.3%	3.1%/1.1%
Finasteride[33]	768/737	4.5%/3.3%	2.4%/1.4%	1.8%/0.8%
Finasteride[59]	1736/579	8.1%/3.8%	5.4%/3.3%	4.0%/0.9%
Finasteride[60]	9423/9457	67.4%/61.5%	65.4%/59.6%	67.4%/61.5%
Finasteride[61]	1524/1516	5.1%/5.1%	2.6%/2.6%	0.2%/0.1%
Finasteride[37]	297/300	3.4%/1.7%	4.7%/1.3%	4.4%/1.7%
Finasteride[62]	310/303	15.8%/6.3%	10%/6.3%	7.7%/1.7%

Open trial data is not included.
Adapted from Welliver C, Butcher M, Potini Y, et al. Impact of alpha blocker, 5-alpha reductase inhibitors and combination therapy on sexual function. Curr Urol Rep 2014;15:441; with permission.

When comparing the reported percentages of sexual side effects experienced while taking either finasteride or dutasteride with those in placebo groups, sexual AEs rates seem to be higher in the medication with a narrowed enzyme target (finasteride). However, in a study with direct comparison of finasteride and dutasteride, side-effect reporting on impotence, decreased libido, EjD, and sexual function disorders were virtually identical.[63] Both finasteride and dutasteride were equally effective in reducing prostate size and improving AUA-Symptom Index (SI) scores, including improvement in Qmax after 12 months of treatment. Another, smaller, study analyzed semen volume following treatment with either finasteride or dutasteride and found ejaculate volumes to be lower than placebo with 21% decrease and 24% decrease in finasteride and dutasteride groups, respectively.[64] A meta-analyses comparison did not find differences with regard to EjD between these 2 medications.[32]

An area of increased concern in the clinical management of patients taking 5ARIs for BPH is the persistence of AE beyond cessation of medication. One study examining the sexual AEs experienced by men taking 5 mg finasteride for 4 years had 4% of the drug group and 2% of the placebo group drop out of the study specifically due to sexual AEs. However, symptom resolution was infrequent in these men, with only 50% of the drug group reporting resolution of symptoms after medication cessation. Interestingly, men in the placebo group who discontinued the study reported symptom resolution in only 41% of cases. It should be noted that in analysis of the PLESS (Proscar Long-Term Efficacy and Safety Study) study, men treated with finasteride experienced new sexual AEs with an increased incidence only during the first year of therapy compared with placebo, once again highlighting a temporal relationship between side-effect severity and therapy course.[65]

Further complicating the association of 5ARIs and sexual dysfunction is the provocative study looking at nocebo or the power of suggestion of sexual AEs and outcomes. In their study, investigators randomized subjects who were starting finasteride treatment to groups who either received no counseling on sexual AEs or were informed that the drug may "cause erectile dysfunction, decreased libido, problems of ejaculation but these are uncommon." The investigators found that there was a significantly higher proportion of sexual dysfunction in the subjects informed of sexual side effects compared with those who were not informed (43.6% vs 15.3%) with increased rates of ED, poor libido, and EjD all reported in the group counseled on sexual AEs.[66]

Combination of 5-Alpha Reductase Inhibitors and Alpha Blockers

A common combination therapy for LUTS due to BPH involves the concomitant use of a 5ARI along with an AB. Examination of study outcomes finds that, although the combination group generally has the best outcomes with regard to urinary symptoms (particularly in groups with the worst symptoms at baseline), the highest rates of sexual AEs also occur in the combination group. However, the larger contributor to the sexual AEs does seem to be the 5ARI and not the AB.

This is evidenced by the MTOPS data in which worsening ED, EjD, and libido were seen in the 5ARI (finasteride) and combination therapy groups (finasteride and doxazosin) but absent from the AB group.[33] In their systematic review and meta-analysis, Gacci and colleagues[32] found EjD was more common with combination therapy than with either ABs (OR = 3.75) or 5ARIs (OR = 2.7) alone. Fwu and colleagues[18] found that combination therapy with doxazosin and finasteride produced the largest deterioration in EjD, erectile function, and overall sexual problems. As mentioned previously, these differences were most pronounced after 1 year of treatment and declined thereafter.

Phosphodiesterase Type 5 Inhibitors

The mechanism by which tadalafil and other phosphodiesterase type 5 inhibitors (PDE5is) provide relief of LUTS due to BPH is still in question. However, available basic science research and expert option hypothesize that the mechanism likely centers on a complex picture of modulation of the autonomic nervous system through NO and cyclic guanosine monophosphate (cGMP) activity. This may decrease prostatic tissue contraction as well as actions, including antiproliferation of prostate and bladder smooth muscle.[67]

Thus far, only a few randomized controlled trials have investigated the efficacy of these medications for LUTS due to BPH, with many more studies demonstrating efficacy with regard to erectile function. For the obvious reasons, sexual AEs are unlikely with PDE5i considering their original indicated use in ED. Tadalafil is currently the

only PDE5i with a dual indication for LUTS due to BPH and ED.

The daily dosing of tadalafil was investigated by Egerdie and colleagues[68] at both the 2.5 mg and 5 mg daily dose. Both doses were well tolerated and, not surprisingly, erectile function scores improved. There were no safety concerns found by the investigators. Although multiple reports have quantified improvements in erectile function with daily tadalafil, few have rigorously examined change in ejaculatory function. In a study using the full IIEF, orgasmic function was also assessed along with ejaculatory frequency and orgasmic frequency. Interestingly, although there was a placebo arm, an active control group taking tamsulosin was included. More than 500 men were examined and improvements were noted in orgasmic function and ejaculatory frequency. Although these are encouraging, this is not the same as augmenting EjD because both of these outcomes could simply be related to an overall improvement in erection quality.[26]

Anticholinergics

Anticholinergics have recently gained popularity as an adjunct therapy in the treatment of men with LUTS due to BPH. Although less frequently used as a first-line medication in men compared with use in women, this medication is commonly used to treat storage symptoms in men once voiding symptoms have been addressed with other medication classes. Anticholinergic medications act by blocking the choline receptor subtypes either in the urothelium or within the detrusor muscle. However, choline or muscarine receptor subtypes are found in multiple other parts of the body and unintended effects such as dry mouth, constipation, tachycardia, and neurologic changes are reported with varying frequency.

Only cursory assessments have been published in the urologic literature regarding the sexual side effects of anticholinergics in men. However, sporadic reports on anticholinergic properties in antidepressant medications demonstrate that provoked sexual dysfunction could be reversed with bethanachol.[69,70]

SURGICAL TREATMENTS
Background

Surgical treatments for LUTS due to BPH may affect sexual function in a variety of ways. EjD may be in the form of retrograde ejaculation by resection of the bladder neck and more proximal portions of the prostate, thus removing the barrier by which the ejaculate is preferentially moved in an antegrade fashion. ED could potentially be induced by overly aggressive treatments that do not respect anatomical planes and injure the adjacent cavernous nerves. In studies looking at increasing ED rates, capsular perforation does seem to predispose men to worsening erectile function.[71] Although effects on libido from surgery are more difficult to connect pathophysiologically, surely any postsurgical incontinence could lead avoidance of sexual situations and reduced libido. Although placebo effects have frequently been studied in medication trials with regard to both urinary outcomes and AEs, surgical BPH treatments have demonstrated a significant sham surgery effect, at least with regard to urinary symptom outcomes.[72]

Transurethral Resection of the Prostate

Transurethral resection of the prostate (TURP) has been the gold standard for surgical treatment of men suffering from LUTS due to BPH for years. Recently, minimally invasive surgical techniques have become increasingly popular,[73] likely due to the decreased associated morbidity.

Ejaculatory dysfunction

The most common side effect experienced by patients who undergo TURP is EjD, primarily in the form of retrograde ejaculation. Studies looking at EjD rates after TURP are sparse but of decent methodological quality because most are done as part of comparative trials. In studies comparing monopolar and bipolar TURP, EjD was in the 50% to 70% range.[74–77] Although this was reproducible across studies, it is likely lower than the real life experience, wherein most providers quote a rate closer to 90% for patients in the preoperative counseling. Although retrograde ejaculation is common, some reports have found an overall improvement in ejaculatory function with TURP because background discomfort or pain associated with ejaculation is relieved.[78]

Erectile dysfunction

TURP is thought to cause ED through a variety of mechanisms but primarily through thermal injury that has spread to the cavernous nerves during surgery. Other potential mechanisms include the psychological effect of surgery and the cessation of sexual activity in the postoperative period. Interestingly, baseline erectile function was compared in a study of subjects undergoing TURP or transurethral resection of the bladder (TURBT). Although the TURBT had better baseline erectile function, the TURP group had improvements in erectile function (improving from 7 to 20 on IIEF-15) with surgical procedure. After TURP, the groups were no longer different with regard to both voiding outcomes and sexual function.[79] These findings are certainly thought-provoking and compliment the theory that LUTS diminishes sexual function.

However, patients may still perceive worsening function with surgery, even when objective data are not in agreement. In their study of more than 500 subjects who underwent TURP, there was a both statistically and clinically insignificant change in IIEF from baseline to 6 month follow-up (18.8 vs 17.8, $P = .79$). However, subject-reported subjective ED increased from 65% to 77%.[71] Affirmingly, in their survey of the Swiss population, Muntener and colleagues[78] found little change in erectile function with the TURP. In studies looking at objective measures or erectile function such as nocturnal penile tumescence,[80] investigators found no loss of function with TURP, and even a small increase in penile rigidity. When men were questioned about their lack of function, 64% associated the new onset retrograde ejaculation with decreased sexual potency.

Although these studies have compared the erectile function of subjects, before and after the procedure, interesting perspective is gained by looking at how erectile function changes are compared with a baseline group on watchful waiting. In the Veterans Affairs cooperative study, men undergoing watchful waiting for LUTS due to BPH were compared with men who underwent TURP. Although this study largely predates ubiquitous medical treatment of BPH, the investigators found that the TURP group had better erectile function than the watchful waiting group at study termination.[81] These findings reinforce the concept of decreasing sexual function with both age and incompletely treated BPH.

Bipolar versus monopolar transurethral resection of the prostate

Monopolar TURP has long been the standard for endoscopic treatments. However, the procedure requires a nonionic irrigating solution that is hypo-osmolar and can be absorbed through the prostatic tissues. When this occurs, patients may become acutely hyponatremic with resulting neurologic repercussions. The advent of the bipolar resection technologies has significantly improved on this concept because resection can now be carried out in iso-osmolar (saline) fluid.

Although benefits have been found with regard to many of the classic BPH study outcomes such as bleeding and catheter times,[76] there are minimal data to support an improvement in sexual outcomes between these different modalities. Although, in theory, the decreased tissue penetration of the bipolar electrocautery could potentially mitigate unintentional cavernous nerve injury and reduce ED rates, this has not been noted in comparative studies to monopolar TURP.[76]

Transurethral Microwave Therapy

Transurethral microwave therapy (TUMT) is a procedure that involves a special catheter that is inserted transurethrally. The catheter acts as an antenna and emits energy that leads to local thermoablation of prostate parenchyma while preserving the bladder neck, external sphincter, and prostatic urothelium. In general, perioperative and postoperative complications are rare, although improvements in voiding outcomes are also generally modest.

With careful temperature monitoring, injury to surrounding structures that would influence sexual function should be rare. Generally, studies evaluating sexual function after TUMT are not rigorous and have not used validated questionnaires. In 1 study, 5% of subjects described new ED.[82] Most studies report low rates of new EjD (less than 5%); however, 1 report noted an unusually high 44% incidence of new EjD.[83] A study surveying subjects on preservation of antegrade ejaculation found 74% of subjects maintained antegrade ejaculation.[84]

Transurethral Needle Ablation

Transurethral needle ablation (TUNA) is similar to TUMT in that it uses a specialized catheter that is inserted per urethra. The TUNA catheter uses 2 prongs that extend into the prostate parenchyma to provide a focal treatment with radiofrequency energy. Again, similar to TUMT, the bladder neck, sphincter, and prostatic urothelium should be largely undisturbed.

In their randomized trial of TURP versus TUNA, Cimentepe and colleagues[85] found no retrograde ejaculation or erection impairment with TUNA. The nonrandomized comparison of TURP, TUNA, and TUMT was less optimistic and found a decrease in erectile function in 18% and 20% of TUMT and TUNA subjects, respectively, with ejaculation loss noted in 28% and 24%.[74]

Prostate Urethral Lift

The prostate urethral lift (PUL) alters the anatomy of the prostate without tissue destruction. The implants are placed via a cystoscope under tension in the lateral or anterolateral aspect of the prostate to compress the prostatic parenchyma and open the urethra. The preservation of the bladder neck minimized EjD and, because the neurovascular bundles running along the prostate are preserved, there should be no change in erectile function.

In 1 of the first studies looking at PUL, 206 men were randomized 2 to 1 to undergo PUL or sham procedure. At 3-month follow-up, AUA-SI improvements were 88% greater in the active treatment group.[86] There was no evidence of sexual dysfunction or EjD with treatment and ejaculatory bother score improved by 40%[87] with minimal changes in sexual function in a subsequent meta-analysis of trials.[88] Recently released 3-year data have demonstrated that improvements in voiding outcomes were durable.[89]

Open Simple Prostatectomy

Although open simple prostatectomy (OP) was a foundation of treatment of BPH for many years, the inherently more invasive nature of the procedure has generally restricted use to large glands (>100 g) in contemporary practice.

Because this is generally an older approach to surgical treatment to BPH, few studies have rigorously studied outcomes with regard to sexual function. In the only study in the literature examining changes in sexual function with OP, 60 men who underwent the procedure were analyzed using validated questionnaires. Results of the IIEF found a decrease in intercourse satisfaction but increases in sexual desire and overall sexual satisfaction.[90]

Holmium Laser Enucleation of the Prostate

The holmium:yttrium-aluminum-garnet (Ho:YAG) has many uses in urology. Although previously used for ablation in BPH, this laser type is now primarily used for enucleation of the prostate lobes in contemporary practice. This technique has a difficult learning curve but has the ability to efficiently treat large glands via an endoscopic approach.

Retrograde ejaculation is seen commonly after holmium laser enucleation of the prostate (HoLEP) with different randomized trials reporting incidence of roughly 75%.[77,91] In a trial comparing TURP to HoLEP, there was no difference in IIEF scores at 7 years postprocedure.[92] Changes in IIEF scores with HoLEP were found to be minimal in another comparative trial.[77]

Photoselective Vaporization of the Prostate

Photoselective vaporization of the prostate (PVP) uses a specialized laser fiber in which wavelength is selectively absorbed by hemoglobin. This allows for vaporization of prostate tissue in a nearly bloodless field. Because the tissue removed is similar to that during TURP, similar outcomes with regard to sexual function after surgery would be expected.

Worsening and improving erections have been demonstrated in cohorts undergoing PVP, although in most cases the changes are modest and generally not clinically significant, even if they are statistically significant.[93–96] Although ejaculation is clearly affected because the bladder neck is frequently vaporized, men still noted an increase in overall sexual satisfaction and a decrease in bother due to sex.[96]

SUMMARY

Innate sexual dysfunction is common in the cohort of men who present to the urologist for treatment of LUTS due to BPH. Although medications and surgeries for BPH may exacerbate these problems, the longitudinal effects of both aging and worsening LUTS may have a large effect on sexual dysfunction. Sexual dysfunction resulting from these treatments is, at best, a secondary outcome in most studies and is infrequently studied rigorously.

REFERENCES

1. Rosen R, Altwein J, Boyle P, et al. Low urinary tract symptoms and male sexual dysfunction: the multinational survey of the aging male (MSAM-7). Eur Urol 2003;44:637–49.
2. Boyle P, Robertson C, Mazzetta C, et al. The association between lower urinary tract symptoms and erectile dysfunction in four centres: the UrEpik study. BJU Int 2003;92:719–25.
3. Braun MH, Sommer F, Haupt G, et al. Lower urinary tract symptoms and erectile dysfunction: co-morbidity or typical "Aging Male" symptoms? Results of the "Cologne Male Survey". Eur Urol 2003;44:588–94.
4. Elliot SP, Gulati M, Pasta DJ, et al. Obstructive lower urinary tract symptoms correlate with erectile dysfunction. Urology 2004;63:1148.
5. Vallancien G, Emberton M, Harving N, et al. Sexual dysfunction in 1,274 European men suffering from lower urinary tract symptoms. J Urol 2003;169: 2257–61.
6. Brookes ST, Donovan JL, Peters TJ, et al. Sexual dysfunction in men after treatment for lower urinary tract symptoms: evidence from randomised controlled trial. BMJ 2002;324:1059–61.
7. Price DT, Schwinn DA, Lomasney JW, et al. Identification, quantification, and localization of mRNA for three distinct alpha 1 adrenergic receptor subtypes in human prostate. J Urol 1993;150:546–51.
8. Smith M, Schambra U, Wilson K, et al. Alpha1-adrenergic receptors in human spinal cord: specific localized expression of mRNA encoding alpha1-adrenergic receptor subtypes at four distinct levels. Brain Res Mol Brain Res 1999;63:254.
9. McVary KT, Roehrborn CG, Avins AL, et al. Update on AUA guideline on the management of benign prostatic hyperplasia. J Urol 2011;185:1793–803.
10. Welliver C, Butcher M, Potini Y, et al. Impact of alpha blocker, 5-alpha reductase inhibitors and combination therapy on sexual function. Curr Urol Rep 2014;15:441.
11. van Kerrebroeck P, Jardin A, Laval KU, et al. Efficacy and safety of a new prolonged release formulation of alfuzosin 10 mg once daily versus alfuzosin 2.5 mg thrice daily and placebo in patients with symptomatic benign prostatic hyperplasia. ALFORTI Study Group. Eur Urol 2000;37:306–13.
12. Andersson KE. The pharmacological perspective: role for the sympathetic nervous system in micturition and sexual function. Prostate Cancer Prostatic Dis 1999;2:S5–8.
13. Nagai A, Hara R, Yokoyama T, et al. Ejaculatory dysfunction caused by the new alpha1-blocker silodosin: a preliminary study to analyze human ejaculation using color Doppler ultrasonography. Int J Urol 2008;15:915–8.
14. Hisasue S, Furuya R, Itoh N, et al. Ejaculatory disorder caused by alpha-1 adrenoceptor antagonists is not retrograde ejaculation but a loss of seminal emission. Int J Urol 2006;13:1311–6.
15. Kobayashi K, Masumori N, Hisasue S, et al. Inhibition of seminal emission is the main cause of anejaculation induced by a new highly selective alpha1A-blocker in normal volunteers. J Sex Med 2008;5:2185–90.
16. Hedlund H, Andersson KE, Larsson B. Effect of drugs interacting with adrenoreceptors and muscarinic receptors in the epididymal and prostatic parts of the human isolated vas deferens. J Auton Pharmacol 1985;5:261–70.
17. Moriyama N, Nasu K, Takeuchi T, et al. Quantification and distribution of alpha 1-adrenoceptor subtype mRNAs in human vas deferens: comparison with those of epididymal and pelvic portions. Br J Pharmacol 1997;122:1009–14.
18. Fwu CW, Eggers PW, Kirkali Z, et al. Change in sexual function in men with lower urinary tract symptoms/benign prostatic hyperplasia associated with long-term treatment with doxazosin, finasteride and combined therapy. J Urol 2013;191(6):1828–34.
19. Kirby RS, Roehrborn C, Boyle P, et al. Efficacy and tolerability of doxazosin and finasteride, alone or in combination, in treatment of symptomatic benign prostatic hyperplasia: the prospective European doxazosin and combination therapy (PREDICT) trial. Urology 2003;61:119–26.
20. van Moorselaar RJ, Hartung R, Emberton M, et al. Alfuzosin 10 mg once daily improves sexual function in men with lower urinary tract symptoms and concomitant sexual dysfunction. BJU Int 2005;95: 603–8.

21. Elhilali M, Emberton M, Matzkin H, et al. ALF-ONE Study Group. Long-term efficacy and safety of alfuzosin 10 mg once daily: a 2-year experience in 'real-life' practice. BJU Int 2006;97:513–9.

22. Höfner K, Claes H, De Reijke TM, et al. Tamsulosin 0.4 mg once daily: effect on sexual function in patients with lower urinary tract symptoms suggestive of benign prostatic obstruction. Eur Urol 1999;36: 335–41.

23. Narayan P, Tewari A. A second phase III multicenter placebo controlled study of 2 dosages of modified release tamsulosin in patients with symptoms of benign prostatic hyperplasia. United States 93-01 Study Group. J Urol 1998;160:1701–6.

24. Shelbaia A, Elsaied WM, Elghamrawy H, et al. Effect of selective alpha-blocker tamsulosin on erectile function in patients with lower urinary tract symptoms due to benign prostatic hyperplasia. Urology 2013;82:130–5.

25. Wilt T, MacDonald R, Rutks I. Tamsulosin for benign prostatic hyperplasia. Cochrane Database Syst Rev 2002;(4):CD002081.

26. Giuliano F, Oelke M, Jungwirth A, et al. Tadalafil once daily improves ejaculatory function, erectile function, and sexual satisfaction in men with lower urinary tract symptoms suggestive of benign prostatic hyperplasia and erectile dysfunction: results from a randomized, placebo- and tamsulosin-controlled, 12-week double-blind study. J Sex Med 2013;10:857–65.

27. Novara G, Chapple CR, Montorsi F. A pooled analysis of individual patient data from registrational trials of silodosin in the treatment of non-neurogenic male lower urinary tract symptoms (LUTS) suggestive of benign prostatic hyperplasia (BPH). BJU Int 2014;114:427–33.

28. Kawabe K, Yoshida M, Homma Y. Silodosin, a new alpha1A-adrenoceptor-selective antagonist for treating benign prostatic hyperplasia: results of a phase III randomized, placebo-controlled, double-blind study in Japanese men. BJU Int 2006;98:1019–24.

29. Hellstrom WJ, Sikka SC. Effects of acute treatment with tamsulosin versus alfuzosin on ejaculatory function in normal volunteers. J Urol 2006;176:1529–33.

30. Karadag E, Oner S, Budak YU, et al. Randomized crossover comparison of tamsulosin and alfuzosin in patients with urinary disturbances caused by benign prostatic hyperplasia. Int Urol Nephrol 2011;43:949–54.

31. Chapple CR, Montorsi F, Tammela TL, et al. Silodosin therapy for lower urinary tract symptoms in men with suspected benign prostatic hyperplasia: results of an international, randomized, double-blind, placebo- and active-controlled clinical trial performed in Europe. Eur Urol 2011;59:342–52.

32. Gacci M, Ficarra V, Sebastianelli A, et al. Impact of medical treatments for male lower urinary tract symptoms due to benign prostatic hyperplasia on ejaculatory function: a systematic review and meta-analysis. J Sex Med 2014;11:1554–66.

33. McConnell JD, Roehrborn CG, Bautista OM, et al. The long-term effect of doxazosin, finasteride, and combination therapy on the clinical progression of benign prostatic hyperplasia. N Engl J Med 2003; 349:2387–98.

34. Marks LS, Gittelman MC, Hill LA, et al. Rapid efficacy of the highly selective alpha(1A)-adrenoceptor antagonist silodosin in men with signs and symptoms of benign prostatic hyperplasia: pooled results of 2 phase 3 studies. J Urol 2013;189:S122–8.

35. Lepor H, Williford WO, Barry MJ, et al. The efficacy of terazosin, finasteride, or both in benign prostatic hyperplasia. Veterans Affairs Cooperative Studies Benign Prostatic Hyperplasia Study Group. N Engl J Med 1996;335:533–9.

36. Okeigwe I, Kuohung W. 5-Alpha reductase deficieny: a 40-year retrospective review. Curr Opin Endocrinol Diabetes Obes 2014;21:483–7.

37. Gormley GJ, Stoner E, Bruskewitz RC, et al. The effect of finasteride in men with benign prostatic hyperplasia. N Engl J Med 1992;327:1185–91.

38. Schirar A, Bonnefond C, Meusnier C, et al. Androgens modulate nitric oxide synthase messenger ribonucleic acid expression in neurons of the major pelvic ganglion in the rat. Endocrinology 1997;138:3093–102.

39. Gur S, Kadowitz PJ, Hellstrom WJ. Effects of 5-alpha reductase inhibitors on erectile function, sexual desire and ejaculation. Expert Opin Drug Saf 2013; 12:81–90.

40. Kunelius P, Lukkarinen O, Hannuksela ML, et al. The effects of transdermal dihydrotestosterone in the aging male: a prospective, randomized, double blind study. J Clin Endocrinol Metab 2002;87: 1467–72.

41. Foresta C, Caretta N, Garolla A, et al. Erectile function in elderly: role of androgens. J Endocrinol Invest 2003;26:77–81.

42. Dubrovsky BO. Steroids, neuroactive steroids and neurosteroids in psychopathology. Prog Neuropsychopharmacol Biol Psychiatry 2005;29:169–92.

43. Belelli D, Lambert JJ. Neurosteroids: endogenous regulators of the GABA(A) receptor. Nat Rev Neurosci 2005;6:565–75.

44. Melcangi RC, Caruso D, Abbiati F, et al. Neuroactive steroid levels are modified in cerebrospinal fluid and plasma of post-finasteride patients showing persistent sexual side effects and anxious/depressive symptomatology. J Sex Med 2013;10:2598–603.

45. Steiner JF. Clinical pharmacokinetics and pharmacodynamics of finasteride. Clin Pharmacokinet 1996;30:16–27.

46. Dörsam J, Altwein J. 5alpha-reductase inhibitor treatment of prostatic diseases: background and

practical implications. Prostate Cancer Prostatic Dis 2009;12:130–6.

47. Roehrborn CG, Boyle P, Nickel JC, et al. Efficacy and safety of a dual inhibitor of 5-alpha-reductase types 1 and 2 (dutasteride) in men with benign prostatic hyperplasia. Urology 2002;60:434–41.

48. Roehrborn CG, Marks LS, Fenter T, et al. Efficacy and safety of dutasteride in the four-year treatment of men with benign prostatic hyperplasia. Urology 2004;63:709–15.

49. Na Y, Ye Z, Zhang S. Efficacy and safety of dutasteride in Chinese adults with symptomatic benign prostatic hyperplasia: a randomized, double-blind, parallel-group, placebo-controlled study with an open-label extension. Clin Drug Investig 2012;32: 29–39.

50. Clark RV, Hermann DJ, Cunningham GR, et al. Marked suppression of dihydrotestosterone in men with benign prostatic hyperplasia by dutasteride, a dual 5a-reductase inhibitor. J Clin Endocrinol Metab 2004;89:2179–84.

51. Debruyne F, Barkin B, van Erps P, et al. Efficacy and safety of the long-term treatment with the dual 5alpha-reductase inhibitor dutasteride in men with symptomatic benign prostatic hyperplasia. Eur Urol 2004;46:488–95.

52. Andriole G, Bostwick DG, Brawley OW, et al. Effect of dutasteride on the risk of prostate cancer. N Engl J Med 2010;362:1192–202.

53. Marberger MJ. Long-term effects of finasteride in patients with benign prostatic hyperplasia: a double-blind, placebo-controlled, multicenter study. PROWESS Study Group. Urology 1998;51:677–86.

54. Kaufman KD, Olsen EA, Whiting D. Finasteride in the treatment of men with androgenetic alopecia. J Am Acad Dermatol 1998;39:578–89.

55. Leyden J, Dunlap F, Miller B, et al. Finasteride in the treatment of men with frontal male pattern hair loss. J Am Acad Dermatol 1999;40:930–7.

56. Whiting DA, Olsen EA, Savin R, et al, Male Pattern Hair Loss Study Group. Efficacy and tolerability of finasteride 1 mg in men aged 41 to 60 years with male pattern hair loss. Eur J Dermatol 2003;13: 150–60.

57. Byrnes CA, Morton AS, Liss CL, et al. Efficacy, tolerability, and effect on health-related quality of life of finasteride versus placebo in men with symptomatic benign prostatic hyperplasia: a community-based study. Clin Ther 1995;17:956–69.

58. Lowe FC, McConnell JD, Hudson PB, et al. Long-term 6-year experience with finasteride in patients with benign prostatic hyperplasia. Urology 2003; 61:791–6.

59. Tenover JL, Pagano GA, Morton AS, et al. Efficacy and tolerability of finasteride in symptomatic benign prostatic hyperplasia: a primary care study. Clin Ther 1997;19:243–58.

60. Thompson IM, Goodman PJ, Tangen CM, et al. The influence of finasteride on the development of prostate cancer. N Engl J Med 2003;349:214–5.

61. McConnell JD, Brusketwitz R, Walsh P, et al. The effect of finasteride on the risk of acute urinary retention and the need for surgical treatment among men with benign prostatic hyperplasia. N Engl J Med 1998; 338:557–63.

62. Nickel J, Curtis MD, Fradet Y, et al. Efficacy and safety of finasteride therapy for benign prostatic hyperplasia: results of a 2-year randomized controlled trial (the PROSPECT study). Can Med Assoc J 1996;155:1251–9.

63. Nickel JC, Gilling P, Tammela TL, et al. Comparison of dutasteride and finasteride for treating benign prostatic hyperplasia: the enlarged prostate international comparator study (EPICS). BJU Int 2011;108: 388–94.

64. Amory JK, Wang C, Swerdloff RS, et al. The effect of 5alpha-reductase inhibition with dutasteride and finasteride on semen parameters and serum hormones in healthy men. J Clin Endocrinol Metab 2007;92:1659–65.

65. Wessels H, Roy J, Bannow J, et al. Incidence and severity of sexual adverse experiences in finasteride and placebo-treated men with benign prostatic hyperplasia. Urology 2003;61:579–84.

66. Mondaini N, Gontero P, Giubilei G, et al. Finasteride 5 mg and sexual side effects: how many of these are related to a nocebo phenomenon? J Sex Med 2007; 4:1708–12.

67. Filippi S, Morelli A, Sandner P, et al. Characterization and functional role of androgen-dependent PDE5 activity in the bladder. Endocrinology 2007;148: 1019–29.

68. Egerdie RB, Auerbach S, Roehrborn CG. Tadalafil 2.5 or 5 mg administered once daily for 12 weeks in men with both erectile dysfunction and signs and symptoms of benign prostatic hyperplasia: results of a randomized, placebo-controlled, double-blind study. J Sex Med 2012;9:271–81.

69. Gross MD. Reversal by bethanechol of sexual dysfunction caused by anticholinergic antidepressants. Am J Psychiatry 1982;139:1193–4.

70. Segraves RT. Reversal by bethanechol of imipramine-induced ejaculatory dysfunction. Am J Psychiatry 1987;144:1243–4.

71. Poulakis B, Ferakis N, Witzsch U, et al. Erectile dysfunction after transurethral prostatectomy for lower urinary tract symptoms: results from a center with over 500 patients. Asian J Androl 2006;8(1): 69–74.

72. Welliver C, Kottwitz M, Feustel P, et al. Clinically and statistically significant changes seen in sham surgery arms of randomized, controlled benign prostatic hyperplasia surgery trials. J Urol 2015;194: 1682–7.

73. Malaeb BS, Yu X, McBean AM, et al. National trends in surgical therapy for benign prostatic hyperplasia in the United States (2000-2008). Urology 2012;79:1111–6.

74. Arai Y, Aoki Y, Okubo K, et al. Impact of interventional therapy for benign prostatic hyperplasia on quality of life and sexual function: a prospective study. J Urol 2000;164:1206–11.

75. Autorino R, De Sio M, D'Armiento M. Bipolar plasma-kinetic technology for the treatment of symptomatic benign prostatic hyperplasia: evidence beyond marketing hype. BJU Int 2007;100:983–5.

76. Issa MM. Technological advances in transurethral resection of the prostate: bipolar versus monopolar TURP. J Endourol 2008;22:1587–95.

77. Briganti A, Naspro R, Gallina A, et al. Impact on sexual function of holmium laser enucleation versus transurethral resection of the prostate: results of a prospective, 2-center, randomized trial. J Urol 2006;175:1817–21.

78. Muntener M, Aellig S, Kuettel R, et al. Sexual function after transurethral resection of the prostate (TURP): results of an independent prospective multi-centre assessment of outcome. Eur Urol 2007;52:510–5.

79. Jaidane M, Arfa NB, Hmida W, et al. Effect of transurethral resection of the prostate on erectile function: a prospective comparative study. Int J Impot Res 2010;22:146–51.

80. Soderdahl DW, Knight RW, Hansberry KL. Erectile dysfunction following transurethral resection of the prostate. J Urol 1996;156:1354.

81. Wasson JH, Reda DJ, Bruskewitz RC, et al. A comparison of transurethral surgery with watchful waiting for moderate symptoms of benign prostatic hyperplasia: the Veterans Affairs Cooperative Study Group on transurethral resection of the prostate. N Engl J Med 1995;332:75.

82. Kirby RS, Williams G, Witherow R, et al. The prostatron transurethral microwave device in the treatment of bladder outflow obstruction due to benign prostatic hyperplasia. Br J Urol 1993;72:190–4.

83. de la Rosette JJ, de Wildt MJ, Hofner K, et al. High energy thermotherapy in the treatment of benign prostatic hyperplasia: results of the European Benign Prostatic Hyperplasia Study Group. J Urol 1996;156:97–101.

84. Francisca EA, d'Ancona FC, Meuleman EJ, et al. Sexual function following high energy microwave thermotherapy: results of a randomized controlled study comparing transurethral microwave thermotherapy to transurethral prostatic resection. J Urol 1999;161:486–90.

85. Cimentepe E, Unsal A, Saglam R. Randomized clinical trial comparing transurethral needle ablation with transurethral resection of the prostate for the treatment of benign prostatic hyperplasia: results at 18 months. J Endourol 2003;17:103–7.

86. Roehrborn CG, Gange SN, Shore ND, et al. The prostatic urethral lift for the treatment of lower urinary tract symptoms associated with prostate enlargement due to benign prostatic hyperplasia: the L.I.F.T. Study. J Urol 2013;190:2161–7.

87. McVary KT, Gange SN, Shore ND, et al. Treatment of LUTS Secondary to BPH while preserving sexual function: randomized controlled study of prostatic urethral lift. J Sex Med 2014;11:279–87.

88. Perera M, Roberts MJ, Doi SA, et al. Prostatic urethral lift improves urinary symptoms and flow while preserving sexual function for men with benign prostatic hyperplasia: a systematic review and meta-analysis. Eur Urol 2015;67:704–13.

89. Roehrborn CG, Rukstalis DB, Barkin J, et al. Three year results of the prostatic urethral L.I.F.T. study. Can J Urol 2015;22:7772–82.

90. Gacci M, Bartoletti R, Figlioli S, et al. Urinary symptoms, quality of life and sexual function in patients with benign prostatic hypertrophy before and after prostatectomy: a prospective study. BJU Int 2003;91:196–200.

91. Wilson LC, Gilling PJ, Williams A, et al. A randomised trial comparing holmium laser enucleation versus transurethral resection in the treatment of prostates larger than 40 grams: results at 2 years. Eur Urol 2006;50:569–73.

92. Gilling PJ, Wilson LC, King CJ, et al. Long-term results of a randomized trial comparing holmium laser enucleation of the prostate and transurethral resection of the prostate: results at 7 years. BJU Int 2011;109:408–11.

93. Paick JS, Um JM, Kim SW, et al. Influence of high-power potassium-titanyl-phosphate photoselective vaporization of the prostate on erectile function: a short-term follow-up study. J Sex Med 2007;4:1701–7.

94. Kavoussi PK, Hermans MR. Maintenance of erectile function after photoselective vaporization of the prostate for obstructive benign prostatic hyperplasia. J Sex Med 2008;5:2669–71.

95. Kumar A, Vasudeva P, Kumar N, et al. A prospective study on the effect of photoselective vaporization of prostate by 120-W high-performance system laser on sexual function. J Endourol 2014;28:1115–20.

96. Terrasa JB, Cornu JN, Haab F, et al. Prospective, multidimensional evaluation of sexual disorders in men after laser photovaporization of the prostate. J Sex Med 2013;10:1363–71.

Testosterone and the Prostate: Artifacts and Truths

Kenneth Jackson DeLay, MD[a], Tobias S. Kohler, MD[b],*

KEYWORDS

• Testosterone • BPH • LUTS • Hypogonadism

KEY POINTS

- Despite a lack of evidence, there have been stated concerns that testosterone replacement therapy (TRT) can pose a risk to men suffering with lower urinary tract symptoms (LUTS)/benign prostatic hyperplasia (BPH).
- TRT may improve components of the metabolic syndrome, which is associated with worsening LUTS. Furthermore, the evidence suggests that TRT may decrease prostatic inflammation, which is also associated with worsening LUTS.
- The data on the relationship between TRT and LUTS have never shown worsening of LUTS, often show no change in LUTS, and occasionally show improvement.

INTRODUCTION

As men age, they tend to become burdened with an increasing number of medical illnesses. Many of these illnesses tend to be urologic. Two of these conditions frequently seen by urologist are hypogonadism and benign prostatic hyperplasia (BPH) with its associated lower urinary tract symptoms (LUTS). Testosterone levels begin decline to in men's middle 30s. Shortly thereafter, many men begin to become bothered by LUTS associated with BPH. Understanding the relationship between LUTS/BPH and hypogonadism is increasingly important, as more aging men inquire about testosterone replacement therapy (TRT).

Several safety concerns have been raised about TRT. In 2015, the FDA required a black box warning regarding a possible increased risk for myocardial infarction and cerebrovascular events. Methods from the studies leading to this conclusion have been called into question.[1,2] Additionally, the US Food and Drug Administration (FDA) issued a black box warning regarding TRT in men with BPH. The warning regarding topical androgens included the following statement:

"Patients with BPH treated with androgens are at an increased risk of worsening of signs and symptoms of BPH. Monitor patients with BPH for worsening signs and symptoms. Patients treated with androgens may be at an increased risk for prostate cancer. Evaluation of patients for prostate cancer prior to initiating and during treatment is appropriate."[3]

The data for these recommendations are unclear, and this article will examine the evidence relating to TRT in men with BPH.

Both hypogonadism and BPH become more prevalent with increasing age in men. This article will examine the pathophysiology leading to both processes and the potential impact of TRT in patients suffering from BPH.

NATURAL HISTORY OF TESTOSTERONE/HYPOGONADISM

Testosterone is the major hormone responsible for male sexual differentiation. It has a short half-life at

[a] Departments of Urology, Tulane University Health Sciences Center, New Orleans, LA, USA; [b] Division of Urology, Southern Illinois University School of Medicine, 301 North 8th Street, 4th Floor, PO Box 19665, Springfield, IL 62794-9665, USA
* Corresponding author.
E-mail address: tkohler@siumed.edu

Urol Clin N Am 43 (2016) 405–412
http://dx.doi.org/10.1016/j.ucl.2016.04.011

12 minutes. Its secretion begins in utero. It is a cholesterol derivative produced in the adrenal and testes that is 98% bound in the blood. It is loosely bound to albumin and binds tightly to sex hormone-binding globulin. Testosterone that is bound to albumin and testosterone that is free is bioavailable. Its release is pulsatile, and its level fluctuates during the day after peaking in the morning.[4] It appears that these fluctuations become less predominant in men over 45 years of age.[5] Peripheral aromatization results in the conversion of androgens to estrogens. Testosterone binds the androgen receptor (AR), which is translocated to the cell nucleus, and results in the production and secretion of peptide growth factors.

In target organs, testosterone undergoes conversion to 5α-dihydrotestosterone (DHT), a more potent androgen, by the enzyme 5α-reductase. There are 3 isoforms of this enzyme. The 5α-reductase inhibitors (5-ARIs) include finasteride and dutasteride. The type 1 isoenzyme exists primarily in the skin and to a lesser extent the prostate. The type 2 isoenzyme is the dominant form in the prostate although present to a lesser extend in the skin and liver.[6] Finasteride inhibits type 2 5-ARI, with dutasteride inhibiting both type 1 and 2 5-ARI. Dutasteride lowers DHT levels to a greater extent than finasteride. These medications have been used to reduce prostatic volume and LUTS.[7,8]

Increasing awareness of late-onset hypogonadism has made it a frequent subject of discussion among physicians and between physicians and their patients. After a plateau in men in their 20s, testosterone levels begin to decline. Additionally, there is an age-related increase in sex hormone-binding globulin decreasing the bioavailable testosterone.[9–15] In a large cross-sectional study, the European Male Aging Study (EMAS), annually there was a 0.4% decline in serum testosterone and a 1.3% decline in free testosterone.[16] There is controversy concerning whether this decline is physiologic or a pathologic process necessitating treatment.[17] Regardless, there has been a global increase in the prescribing of TRT.[18]

The diagnosis of hypogonadism requires a combination of clinical symptoms and biochemical evidence. There are specific and nonspecific symptoms. Signs and symptoms include: low libido, decrease in muscle mass, anemia, fatigue, decrease in erections, low bone mineral density, and dysthymia. The Androgen Deficiency in Aging Males (ADAM) questionnaire can be helpful in ascertaining this information.[19,20] The Endocrine Society Guidelines published in 2010 do not recommend routine screening.[21] Testing for hypogonadism should consist of a morning total testosterone. A patient with a total testosterone less than 250 is likely to have hypogonadism and should be treated accordingly. Patients with a total T between 250 and 400 should undergo further testing for a free testosterone. Patients with a total testosterone of more than 400 are unlikely to have hypogonadism.[22]

There is no causal link between testosterone therapy and an increased incidence of prostate cancer or LUTS associated with BPH; however, both the International Society of Andrology and the Endocrine society recommend against exogenous testosterone therapy in men who have significant LUTS prior to a urologic evaluation.[23]

NATURAL HISTORY OF BENIGN PROSTATIC HYPERPLASIA

BPH is a technically a histologic diagnosis characterized by the proliferation of prostatic epithelial and stromal cells in the transition zone. Most commonly the diagnosis is made based on clinical symptoms and less commonly radiographic images. Androgen stimulation is required for fetal prostate development. The prostate is small at birth, approximately 1.5 g, and remains stable at this size until puberty. At puberty the gland reaches approximately 10 g. Typically, a prostate reaches its normal weight of 20 g between 21 and 30 years of age.[24] In autopsy studies, the incidence of histologic BPH increases with age, being present in 8% of men 31 to 40 years of age, 42% of those 51 to 60 years of age, and 90% of those older than 90.[25] BPH itself is associated with both erectile and ejaculatory dysfunction. Although contributory, the obstructive effect of hyperplastic nodules does not provide sufficient explanation for the LUTS associated with BPH.

Androgens are necessary but not sufficient for the development of BPH. Animal studies have helped elucidate this role. In a canine study, young castrated dogs only developed BPH after testosterone replacement. BPH regressed in older dogs after the castration but returned following exogenous testosterone administration.[26] Men with primary hypogonadism, who normally do not develop BPH, can now develop BPH after TRT.[27]

Obesity and the metabolic syndrome are both risk factors for LUTS associated with BPH. Obesity is a risk factor for hypogonadism as well. A cross-sectional study examining 100 men with moderate and severe obesity found a negative correlation between androgens (both testosterone/free testosterone) and insulin resistance.[28] It is also interesting to note that multiple studies have demonstrated improvement in hypogonadism after weight loss secondary to bariatric surgery.[29] TRT also is conducive to weight loss.[30] Hyperinsulinemia is associated with increased sympathetic nervous system activity, which may affect smooth muscle tone in the prostate and thus worsen LUTS independent of the obstruction associated with macronodular hyperplasia.[31,32] The metabolic syndrome also creates a proinflammatory milieu within the prostate, which ultimately leads to epithelial and stromal proliferation. In addition patients with the metabolic syndrome have increased amounts of body fat, which leads to the aromatization of androgens into estrogens, further worsening hypogonadism. Studies have established that in conjunction with DHT, estrogen leads to an increase in prostate weight.[33]

Multiple studies have demonstrated an increase in the severity of LUTS in men with the metabolic syndrome. The NHANES III study, an observational study with 2732 men, found an 80% increase in the incidence of LUTS in those with 3 or more components MetS compared to those with none.

The Baltimore Longitudinal Study on Aging demonstrated that for each 1 kg/m^2 increase in body mass index (BMI) there was a 0.41 mL increase in prostatic volume; thus in this study obese men had a 3.5-fold increased risk for an enlarged prostate compared with non-obese men.[34] This is further corroborated by a subsequent paper from this study showing that in radical prostatectomy specimens there was a 0.45 g increase in weight for each additional 1 kg/m^2 increase in BMI.[35]

ANDROGENS AND THEIR INTERACTION WITH BENIGN PROSTATIC HYPERPLASIA

Significant LUTS/BPH is often considered a relative contraindication to TRT. This is based on the pathophysiology connecting androgens to prostatic development and growth. There has been some controversy concerning the impact of TRT on LUTS and related quality of life. This continues to generate concern. There are multiple reasons to suspect that TRT would not have an adverse effect on LUTS and BPH. The first is that the prostate's androgen receptor appears to saturate above a testosterone level of 50 ng/mL; therefore changes in testosterone levels after TRT would not affect the majority of hypogonadal men.[36] Second the intraprostatic levels of androgens do not appear to mirror serum levels.[37,38] In a double-blind, placebo-controlled randomized controlled trial (RCT) by Page and colleagues,[38] patients were randomized to either transdermal DHT or placebo. At 4 weeks of follow-up, there was no difference in either DHT or testosterone between the 2 arms.

The decline of testosterone levels and growth of prostatic tissue are often concurrent processes in the aging man. Prostate growth increases over time, while testosterone levels decline.[25] Data

from the Olmsted County study have shown that lower bioavailable testosterone and rapidly declining testosterone levels are associated with prostatic growth.[39]

There are several questions regarding the impact of TRT on patients with BPH. Principally, does TRT have an impact on prostate volume? To answer this question a randomized control (44 hypogonadal men with moderate-to-severe LUTS) was treated with injectable testosterone enthanate for 6 months. This study did not demonstrate any significant change in prostate volume as measured by magnetic resonance imaging. Additionally, prostate biopsies did not demonstrate a change in tissue testosterone levels.[40] Another randomized double-blind, placebo-controlled trial from the Netherlands with 237 men randomized to either testosterone undeconoate versus placebo showed no change in prostate volume as measured by transrectal ultrasound after 6 months[41] with a similar study from Moscow demonstrating similar findings.[42] It is important to note that changes in prostate volume were not the primary end point in these trials, and thus they may not have been adequately powered to detect a difference.

Multiple cohort studies of hypogonadal men undergoing TRT did not demonstrate an increase in prostate volume.[43–45] A prospective cohort of 25 patients receiving testosterone undeconoate showed a statistically significant increase, although modest, in prostate volume after 12 months of therapy going from a mean of 19.7 to 22 mL.[46] It is worth noting that there was no further increase in prostate volume after a total of 4 years of follow up.

Secondary, how does TRT affect LUTS in those with BPH? In the double blind-placebo controlled trial by Emmelot-Von and colleagues[41] men treated testosterone undeconoate did not show any change in International Prostate Symptom Score (IPSS) at 6 months of follow up. Another randomized trial with transdermal testosterone showed no statistically significant change in IPSS after 12 months of therapy.[47] A randomized study by Tan and colleagues[48] with patients receiving injectable testosterone showed a trend towards improvement in IPSS that did not reach statistical significance. A randomized nonblinded study by Shigehara and colleagues[49] even showed a statistically significant improvement in IPSS and maximal flow rate in those treated with injectable testosterone. Multiple open-label observation studies have shown improvement in IPSS scores after treatment with TRT.[50,51] Consistent with this treatment of hypogonadism of improved voiding status in a trial by Karazindiyanoglu and

Table 1
Outcomes of studies assessing the effect of TRT on the Prostate/LUTS

Study	Location	# of Patients	Follow-up	Design	Data Followed	Therapy	Outcomes
Emmelot-Vonk et al,[41] 2008	The Netherlands	207	6 mo	RCT, double-blind, placebo-controlled	Prostate volume measured by TRUS, PSA, IPSS	IM Testosterone Undecanoate vs placebo	No increase in TRUS volume with TRT No change in IPSS or PSA
Kalinchenko et al,[42] 2010	Russia	184	30 wk	RCT, double-blind, placebo-controlled	IPSS	IM Testosterone Undecanoate vs placebo	No change in IPSS
Haider et al,[44] 2009	Multinational	122	24 mo	Prospectively Followed cohort	IPSS	IM Testosterone Undecanoate vs placbo	Decrease in IPSS with TU treatment ($P<.05$)
Kenny et al,[47] 2010	United States	27	3 mo	Prospective Open-label study	IPSS	Transdermal testosterone	No change in IPSS with TRT
Tan et al,[48] 2013	Malaysia	114	48 wk	RCT, double-blind, placebo-controlled	IPSS	IM Testosterone Undecanoate vs placebo	No Change in IPSS with TRT
Shigehara et al,[49] 2011	Japan	46	12 mo	RCT with untreated control group	IPSS Qmax PVR Prostate volume	IM Testosterone Enthanate vs placebo	Decrease in IPSS & Qmax with TRT ($P<.05$)
Saad et al,[50] 2007	Germany	28	12 mo	Prospective Uncontrolled	IPSS	IM Testosterone Undecanoate vs Transdermal testosterone	Both arms Demonstrated a decrease in IPSS compared to baseline ($P = .05$)
Yassin et al,[51] 2014	Germany	152	5.5 y	Prospective Uncontrolled Registry study	IPSS	IM Testosterone Undecanoate	Decrease in IPSS from 10.35 to 6.31 with no statistical analysis
Karazindiyaoğlu et al,[52] 2008	Turkey	25	12 mo	Prospective cohort study	IPSS, bladder compliance, maximal bladder capacity	Transdermal testosterone	Increase in bladder capacity and compliance with TRT ($P<.05$).

Note: There are no trials showing an increasing in IPSS scores.
Abbreviations: IM, intramuscular; TRUS, transrectal ultrasound.

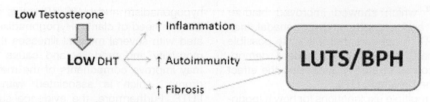

Fig. 1. Relationship of low T/DHT to LUTS/BPH.

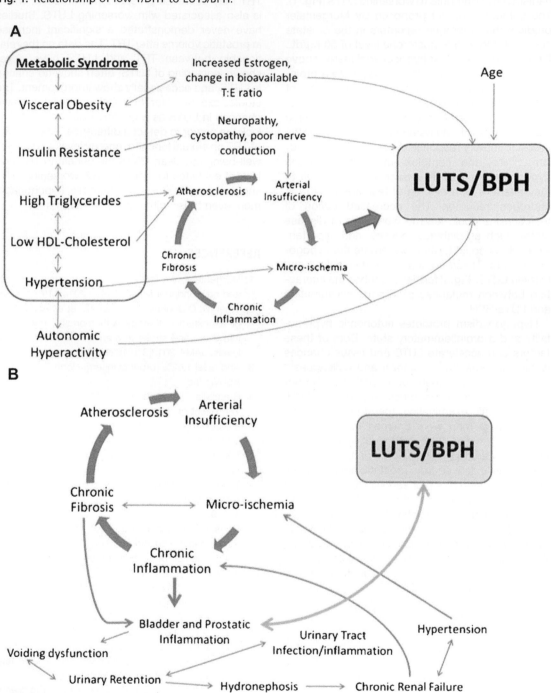

Fig. 2. Interaction between metabolic syndrome, inflammation, and LUTS/BPH. (*A*) Metabolic Syndrome. (*B*) Cardiovascular Disease.

colleagues[52] which showed improved bladder compliance and capacity in hypogonadal men receiving TRT. It appears that it is quite possible that TRT may improve LUTS. **Table 1** demonstrates outcomes of studies assessing the effect of TRT on the prostate/LUTS.

There are multiple explanations for how hypogonadism may contribute to worsening LUTS (**Fig. 1**). The saturation model proposed by Morgentaler predicts that androgen receptors in the prostate are saturated at a testosterone level of 50 ng/dL. First, it is possible that hypogonadal states above a testosterone of 50 ng/dL contribute to a proinflammatory state in the prostate. Second, different organs may have different saturation levels for testosterone; therefore other systems may need higher levels of testosterone to attenuate the proinflammatory response caused by hypogonadism. Third, the complex interaction between hypogonadism and its associated comorbidities may interfere with binding of testosterone to the androgen receptor. The decreased action of testosterone could lead to worsening of disease states such as diabetes, obesity, and hypertension, which could further exacerbate the hypogonadal state. These comorbidities themselves can worsen LUTS. **Fig. 2** further describes the interaction between metabolic syndrome, inflammation and LUTs/BPH.

Hypogonadism promotes autonomic hyperactivity and a proinflammatory state. Both of these factors can accelerate LUTS and tissue changes within the prostate.[53] Vignozzi and colleagues[54] examined the specimens of 42 patients who underwent a suprapubic prostatectomy for BPH. On pathologic examination, the study found that hypogonadal men were 5 times more likely to have inflammation than eugonadal men. Furthermore, they found that in cultured human prostatic stromal cells derived from prostatic adenoma, the potent androgen receptor agonist DHT decreased the release of proinflammatory cytokines.

There is a clear association between worsening LUTS/BPH and increasing sexual dysfunction (both erectile dysfunction and ejaculatory dysfunction),[55] and 18.5% to 23% of men with hypogonadism will have erectile dysfunction that is frequently responsive to TRT.[56,57]

SUMMARY

Despite a lack of evidence, there have been stated concerns that TRT can pose a risk to men suffering with LUTS/BPH. It is clear that prostatic development is dependent upon androgens, although androgens are certainly not the only driver of BPH. Given the large number of men with both hypogonadism and LUTS/BPH, this presents an issue in need of clarity. Hypogonadism is associated with several medical illnesses that increase morbidity and mortality and cause LUTS. TRT may improve components of the metabolic syndrome, which is associated with worsening LUTS. Furthermore, the evidence suggests that TRT may decrease prostatic inflammation, which is also associated with worsening LUTS. Studies have never demonstrated a significant increase in prostatic volume after TRT. The data on the relationship between TRT and LUTS have never shown worsening of LUTS, often show no change in LUTS, and occasionally show improvement. The studies examined for this relationship did not have changes in LUTS as a primary outcome and may lack the power to detect a difference. The benefits of TRT on sexual function, energy level, and overall well-being are clear. Given the benefit to TRT and lack of evidence for risk of LUTS worsening, TRT should be offered to symptomatic hypogonadal men, even those with urinary symptoms.

REFERENCES

1. Morgentaler A. Testosterone, cardiovascular risk, and hormonophobia. J Sex Med 2014;11(6):1362–6.
2. Vigen R, O'Donnell CI, Barón AE, et al. Association of testosterone therapy with mortality, myocardial infarction, and stroke in men with low testosterone levels. JAMA 2013;310:1829–36.
3. AndroGel 1.62% [product insert]. North Chicago, IL: AbbVie Inc.
4. Brambilla DJ, Matsumoto AM, Araujo AB, et al. The effect of diurnal variation on clinical measurement of serum testosterone and other sex hormone benign prostatic hyperplasia levels in men. J Clin Endocrinol Metab 2009;94(3):907–13.
5. Welliver RC Jr, Wiser HJ, Brannigan RE, et al. Validity of midday total testosterone levels in older men with erectile dysfunction. J Urol 2014;192(1): 165–9.
6. Bartsch G, Rittmaster RS, Klocker H. Dihydrotestosterone and the concept of 5α-reductase inhibition in human benign prostatic hyperplasia. Eur Urol 2000; 37:367–80.
7. Gormley GJ, Stoner E, Bruskewitz RC, et al. The effect of finasteride in men with benign prostatic hyperplasia. N Engl J Med 1992;327:1185–91.
8. Roehrborn CG, Boyle P, Nickel JC, et al. Efficacy and safety of a dual inhibitor of 5α-reductase types 1 and 2 (dutasteride) in men with benign prostatic hyperplasia. Urology 2002;60:434–41.
9. Araujo AB, Esche GR, Kupelian V, et al. Prevalence of symptomatic androgen deficiency in men. J Clin Endocrinol Metab 2007;92(11):4241–7.

10. Gapstur SM, Gann PH, Kopp P, et al. Serum androgen concentrations in young men: a longitudinal analysis of associations with age, obesity, and race. The CARDIA male hormone study. Cancer Epidemiol Biomarkers Prev 2002;11(10 Pt 1):1041–7.

11. Gray A, Feldman HA, McKinlay JB, et al. Age, disease, and changing sex hormone levels inmiddle-aged men: results of the Massachusetts Male Aging Study. J Clin Endocrinol Metab 1991; 73(5):1016–25.

12. Harman SM, Metter EJ, Tobin JD, et al. Longitudinal effects of aging on serum total and free testosterone levels in healthy men. Baltimore Longitudinal Study of Aging. J Clin Endocrinol Metab 2001;86(2):724–31.

13. Liu PY, Beilin J, Meier C, et al. Age-related changes in serum testosterone and sex hormone binding globulin in Australian men: longitudinal analyses of two geographically separate regional cohorts. J Clin Endocrinol Metab 2007;92(9): 3599–603.

14. Morley JE, Kaiser FE, Perry HM 3rd, et al. Longitudinal changes in testosterone, luteinizing hormone, and follicle-stimulating hormone in healthy older men. Metabolism 1997;46(4):410–3.

15. Zmuda JM, Cauley JA, Kriska A, et al. Longitudinal relation between endogenous testosterone and cardiovascular disease risk factors in middle-aged men. A 13-year followup of former multiple risk factor intervention trial participants. Am J Epidemiol 1997; 146(8):609–17.

16. Wu FC, Tajar A, Pye SR, et al. Hypothalamic-pituitary-testicular axis disruptions in older men are differentially linked to age and modifiable risk factors: the European Male Aging Study. J Clin Endocrinol Metab 2008;93(7):2737–45.

17. Basaria S. Testosterone therapy in older men with late-onset hypogonadism: a counter-rationale. Endocr Pract 2013;19(5):853–63.

18. Handelsman DJ. Global trends in testosterone prescribing, 2000-2011: expanding the spectrum of prescription drug misuse. Med J Aust 2013;199(8): 548–51.

19. Morley JE, Charlton E, Patrick P, et al. Validation of a screening questionnaire for androgen deficiency in aging males. Metabolism 2000;49(9):1239–42.

20. Morley JE, Perry HM 3rd, Kevorkian RT, et al. Comparison of screening questionnaires for the diagnosis of hypogonadism. Maturitas 2006;53(4): 424–9.

21. Bhasin S, Cunningham GR, Hayes FJ, et al. Testosterone therapy in men with androgen deficiency syndromes: an Endocrine Society clinical practice guideline. J Clin Endocrinol Metab 2010;95(6): 2536–59.

22. Bhasin S, Basaria S. Diagnosis and treatment of hypogonadism in men. Best Pract Res Clin Endocrinol Metab 2011;25(2):251–70.

23. Wang C, Nieschlag E, Swerdloff R, et al. Investigation, treatment, and monitoring of late onset hypogonadism in males: ISA, ISSAM, EAU, EAA, and ASA recommendations. Eur Urol 2009;55(1): 121–30.

24. Vignozzi L, Rastrelli G, Corona G, et al. Benign prostatic hyperplasia: a new metabolic disease? J Endocrinol Invest 2014;37(4):313–22.

25. Berry SJ, Coffey DS, Walsh PC, et al. The development of human benign prostatic hyperplasia with age. J Urol 1984;132(3):474–9.

26. Berry SJ, Coffey DS, Strandberg JD, et al. Effect of age, castration, and testosterone replacement on the development and restoration of canine benign prostatic hyperplasia. Prostate 1986;9:295–302.

27. Sasagawa I, Nakada T, Kazama T, et al. Volume change of the prostate and seminal vesicles in male hypogonadism after androgen replacement therapy. Int Urol Nephrol 1990;22:279–84.

28. Calderón B, Gómez-Martín JM, Vega-Piñero B, et al. Prevalence of male secondary hypogonadism in moderate to severe obesity and its relationship with insulin resistance and excess body weight. Andrology 2016;4(1):62–7.

29. Pellitero S, Olaizola I, Alastrue A, et al. Hypogonadotropic hypogonadism in morbidly obese males is reversed after bariatric surgery. Obes Surg 2012; 22(12):1835–42.

30. Traish AM. Testosterone and weight loss: the evidence. Curr Opin Endocrinol Diabetes Obes 2014; 21(5):313–22.

31. Rohrmann S, Smith E, Giovannucci E, et al. Association between markers of the metabolic syndrome and lower urinary tract symptoms in the Third National Health and Nutrition Examination Survey (NHANES III). Int J Obes (Lond) 2005;29:310–6.

32. Sarma AV, Parsons JK, McVary K, et al. Diabetes and benign prostatic hyperplasia/lower urinary tract symptoms—what do we know? J Urol 2009;182: S32–7.

33. Coffey DS. Similarities of prostate and breast cancer: evolution, diet, and estrogens. Urology 2001;57:31–8.

34. Parsons JK, Carter HB, Partin AW, et al. Metabolic factors associated with benign prostatic hyperplasia. J Clin Endocrinol Metab 2006;91:2562–8.

35. Kopp RP, Ham M, Partin AW, et al. Obesity and prostate enlargement in men with localized prostate cancer. BJU Int 2011;108:1750–5.

36. Morgentaler A, Traish AM. Shifting the paradigm of testosterone and prostate cancer: the saturation model and the limits of androgen-dependent growth. Eur Urol 2009;55(2):310–20.

37. Page ST, Lin DW, Mostaghel EA, et al. Persistent intraprostatic androgen concentrations after medical castration in healthy men. J Clin Endocrinol Metab 2006;91(10):3850–6.

38. Page ST, Lin DW, Mostaghel EA, et al. Dihydrotestosterone administration does not increase intraprostatic androgen concentrations or alter prostate androgen action in healthy men: a randomized-controlled trial. J Clin Endocrinol Metab 2011; 96(2):430–7.

39. St Sauver JL, Jacobson DJ, McGree ME, et al. Associations between longitudinal changes in serum estrogen, testosterone, and bioavailable testosterone and changes in benign urologic outcomes. Am J Epidemiol 2011;173(7):787–96.

40. Marks LS, Mazer NA, Mostaghel E, et al. Effect of testosterone replacement therapy on prostate tissue in men with late-onset hypogonadism: a randomized controlled trial. JAMA 2006;296:2351–61.

41. Emmelot-vonk MH, Verhaar HJ, Nakhai Pour HR. Effect of testosterone supplementation on functional mobility, cognition, and other parameters in older men. JAMA 2008;299:39–52.

42. Kalinchenko SY, Tishova YA, Mskhalaya GJ, et al. Effects of testosterone supplementation on markers of the metabolic syndrome and inflammation in hypogonadal men with the metabolic syndrome: the double-blinded placebo-controlled Moscow study. Clin Endocrinol (Oxf) 2010;73:602–12.

43. Haider A, Gooren LJG, Padungtod P, et al. A safety study of administration of parenteral testosterone undecanoate to elderly men over minimally 24 months. Andrologia 2010;42:349–55.

44. Haider A, Gooren LJ, Padungtod P, et al. Concurrent improvement of the metabolic syndrome and lower urinary tract symptoms upon normalisation of plasma testosterone levels in hypogonadal elderly men. Andrologia 2009;41:7–13.

45. Yassin AA, Saad F. Improvement of sexual function in men with late onset hypogonadism treated with testosterone only. J Sex Med 2007;4:497–501.

46. Minnemann T, Schubert M, Hübler D, et al. A four-year efficacy and safety study of the long-acting parenteral testosterone undecanoate. Aging Male 2007;10:155–8.

47. Kenny AM, Kleppinger A, Annis K, et al. Effects of transdermal testosterone on bone and muscle in older men with low bioavailable testosterone levels, low bone mass, and physical frailty. J Gerontol A Biol Sci Med Sci 2010;56:1134–43.

48. Tan WS, Low WY, Ng CJ, et al. Efficacy and safety of long-acting intramuscular testosterone undecanoate in aging men: a randomised controlled study. BJU Int 2013;111:1130–40.

49. Shigehara K, Sugimoto K, Konaka H, et al. Androgen replacement therapy contributes to improving lower urinary tract symptoms in patients with hypogonadism and benign prostate hypertrophy: a randomised controlled study. Aging Male 2011;14:53–8.

50. Saad F, Gooren L, Haider A, et al. An exploratory study of the effects of 12 month administration of the novel long-acting testosterone undecanoate on measures of sexual function and the metabolic syndrome. Syst Biol Reprod Med 2007;53:353–7.

51. Yassin D-J, Doros G, Hammerer PG, et al. Long-term testosterone treatment in elderly men with hypogonadism and erectile dysfunction reduces obesity parameters and improves metabolic syndrome and health-related quality of life. J Sex Med 2014;11: 1567–76.

52. Karazindiyanoğlu S, Cayan S. The effect of testosterone therapy on lower urinary tract symptoms/bladder and sexual functions in men with symptomatic late-onset hypogonadism. Aging Male 2008;11: 146–9.

53. McVary KT, Rademaker A, Lloyd GL, et al. Autonomic nervous system overactivity in men with lower urinary tract symptoms secondary to benign prostatic hyperplasia. J Urol 2005;174(4 Pt 1):1327–433.

54. Vignozzi L, Cellai I, Santi R, et al. Antiinflammatory effect of androgen receptor activation in human benign prostatic hyperplasia cells. J Endocrinol 2012;214(1):31–43.

55. Rosen R, Altwein J, Boyle P, et al. Lower urinary tract symptoms and male sexual dysfunction: The multinational survey of the aging male (MSAM-7). Eur Urol 2003;44:637–49.

56. Bodie J, Lewis J, Schow D, et al. Laboratory evaluations of erectile dysfunction: an evidence based approach. J Urol 2003;169(6):2262–4.

57. Kohler TS, Kim J, Feia K, et al. Prevalence of androgen deficiency in men with erectile dysfunction. Urology 2008;71(4):693–7.

Index

Note: Page numbers of article titles are in **boldface** type.

urologic.theclinics.com

Moving?

Make sure your subscription moves with you!

To notify us of your new address, find your **Clinics Account Number** (located on your mailing label above your name), and contact customer service at:

Email: journalscustomerservice-usa@elsevier.com

800-654-2452 (subscribers in the U.S. & Canada)
314-447-8871 (subscribers outside of the U.S. & Canada)

Fax number: 314-447-8029

Elsevier Health Sciences Division
Subscription Customer Service
3251 Riverport Lane
Maryland Heights, MO 63043

*To ensure uninterrupted delivery of your subscription, please notify us at least 4 weeks in advance of move.

Printed and bound by CPI Group (UK) Ltd, Croydon, CR0 4YY

22/10/2024

01777562-0001